Move
Without
Pain

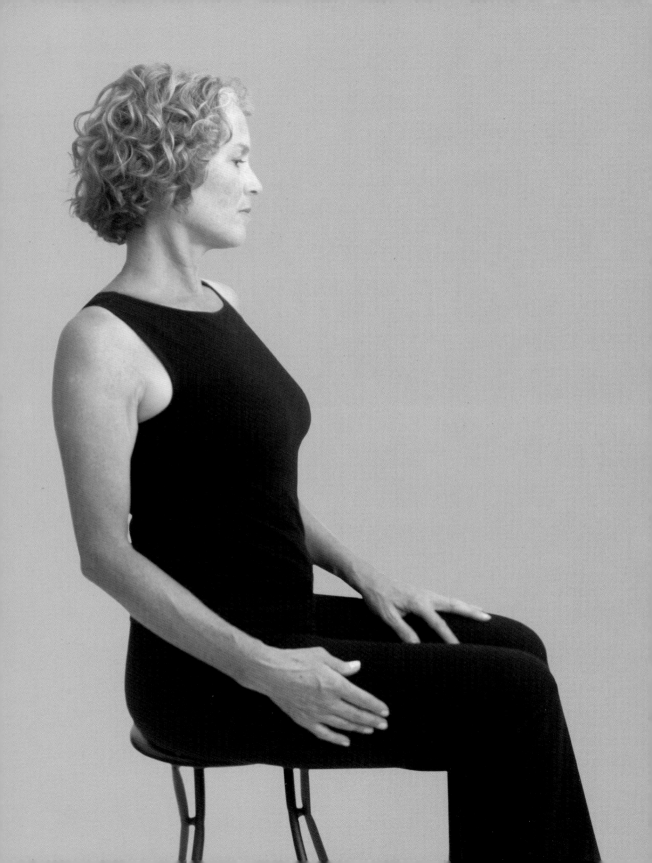

Move Without Pain

Martha Peterson

Photographs by Natalie Galante

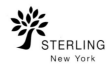

STERLING
New York

STERLING
New York

An Imprint of Sterling Publishing
387 Park Avenue South
New York, NY 10016

ISBN 978-1-4027-7459-1 (paperback)
ISBN 978-1-4027-9087-4 (ebook)

Distributed in Canada by Sterling Publishing
C/o Canadian Manda Group, 165 Dufferin Street
Toronto, Ontario, Canada M6K 3H6
Distributed in the United Kingdom by GMC Distribution Services
Castle Place, 166 High Street, Lewes, East Sussex, England BN7 1XU
Distributed in Australia by Capricorn Link (Australia) Pty. Ltd.
P.O. Box 704, Windsor, NSW 2756, Australia

Book design and layout: *tabula rasa* graphic design

For information about custom editions, special sales, and premium and
corporate purchases, please contact Sterling Special Sales at 800-805-5489
or specialsales@sterlingpublishing.com.

Manufactured in China

8 10 9

www.sterlingpublishing.com

Medical disclaimer: Information contained in this book is intended as an educational
aid only. It is not intended as medical advice, nor does it replace the need for services
provided by medical professionals. The reader is encouraged to consult a physician
before beginning any new regimen of movement. The author and publisher expressly
disclaim any responsibility for any unforeseen circumstances resulting from the use of
any information or instruction contained in this book.

To Thomas Hanna,

whose insights have changed my life

Contents

Part III: Taking the Next Steps 139

Acknowledgments

Awareness isn't something that happens in a vacuum. Self-awareness teaches us how to navigate life, overcome adversity, and move to the next step—if we pay attention, that is. We develop self-awareness through our interactions with others, which also hopefully sheds light on our motivation, our core values, and what really matters to us. We often achieve our goals only because the people who care about us nudge us, push us, and even annoy us to such an extent that we finally take action. I am deeply grateful to many people for having been such a catalyst for me.

I could not have written this book without the support of my special friends—those who could have given me twenty reasons why I shouldn't write a book but didn't. Instead, they stood by to help in any way they could. Thanks to them all, including Ed Myers, who jump-started this project and listened with enthusiasm as I, a nonwriter, explained my idea for this book. His generosity in sharing his knowledge took the fear and angst out of the entire process.

Thanks also to my teachers Marilyn Warnock and Karen Hewitt, who taught me everything they learned from Thomas Hanna, holding nothing back. They helped me to become the practitioner that I am today. Thanks to Ed Barrera, who worked with my sister many years ago. Had it not been for his excellent work, I might never have been exposed to the work of Thomas Hanna when I needed it most. Chris Lowndes helped improve this book with his careful reading of my first draft and his constant reminder to "keep it simple, stupid!" He's always there with humor, to challenge my brain with new ideas and new ways of thinking, moving, and creating. Thank you to Frank

Forencich for his insights into how to be primal, practical, and playful. Thank you to my mother, Meg Peterson, whose example keeps me on my toes and inspires me to never stop moving.

Many thanks to those at Sterling Publishing who made it all happen, including Jennifer Williams and Michael Fragnito—what a nice bunch of people! Thank you to Edward Ash-Milby of Barnes & Noble, and to Barbara Clark for her manuscript editing.

Finally, thank you to members of my tribe: Louise Vitello, for her enthusiastic support of somatics; Cheryl Galante, for keeping me thinking big; Carrie Day, for teaching this important work; my sister, Cary Peterson, for having told me about Hanna Somatics many years ago; Natalie Galante, for her photography; and my husband, Gary Shippy, who gave me a shot in the arm and some excellent feedback when I most needed it. Thank you all.

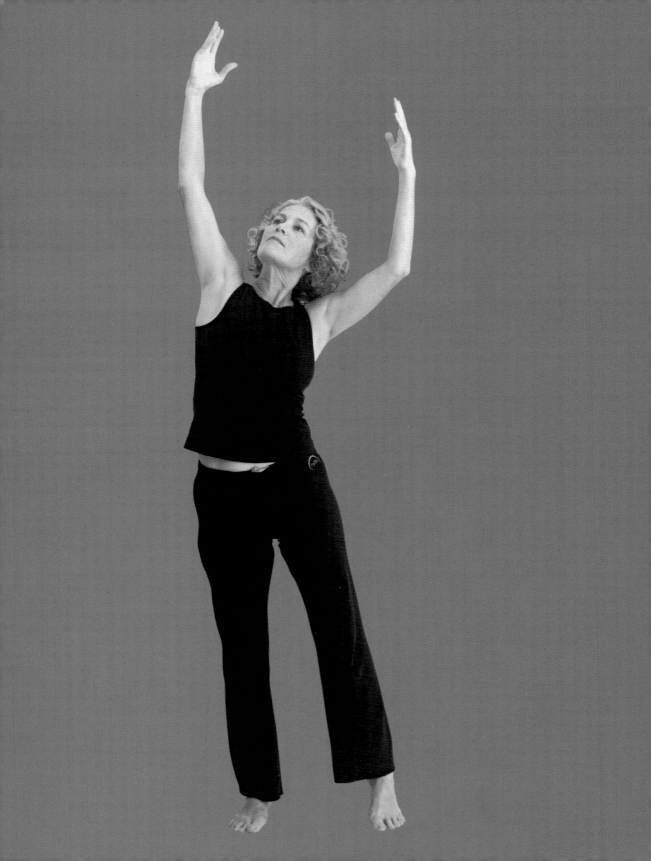

PART I

Preparing to Move Without Pain

The "Mystery" of Muscular Pain

We live in the twenty-first century, in a developed country that is obsessed with the importance of an attractive body and rigorous physical exercise. Never before has the United States seen such a proliferation of personal trainers, gym memberships, fitness TV shows, innovations in exercise equipment, and books on "staying young." Just go to your local bookstore and check out the section on personal fitness. The selection is daunting. Moreover, the vast majority of us do not begin the quest for a healthier life with a full understanding of how the body, muscles, and mind can work together in order to produce the best results. We need a clear and practical method for reconnecting our minds with our bodies so that we can eliminate pain and improve our overall health.

Despite the popularity of exercise, fitness books, and diet programs, the fact remains that there are increasing numbers of people, both young and old, complaining of chronic muscular pain. Painkillers take up entire walls of the local drugstore, catering to myriad new pain symptoms that crop up seemingly daily. Younger and younger amateur athletes and "weekend warriors" wind up in the doctor's office suffering from muscle strain as well as overuse and overtraining injuries. Their desire to be fit and active is well-intentioned, but their techniques are apparently doing them more harm than good. I hear more and more people saying "It's probably just my age" when discussing their pain. Much of this pain is preventable—and reversible—when one understands the physiology behind many common cases of chronic pain and what can be done to end it.

According to a 2008 article in the *Journal of the American Medical Association*, the cost of treating back pain alone has risen to $85.9 billion! More disturbing was the accompanying quote by a health policy expert from the University of Washington: "We are putting a lot more money into this problem and not seeing any improvement in health." Why is this? Is it that back pain and other kinds of muscular pain are really so mysterious, or are most people looking for the solution without having first asked an important question: "How do muscles become tight in the first place?"

This book is about unlocking the "mystery" of muscular pain. It is based upon the discoveries of Thomas Hanna, PhD (1928–1990), who combined his expertise in philosophy, movement education, and neurophysiology to create Hanna Somatic Education (also known as Clinical Somatic Education). As a philosopher, he understood that humans have a capacity for intellectual freedom. As a movement educator, practicing the work of Moshe Feldenkrais, he understood that humans have an ability to become more self-sensing and in control of their lives. His studies in neurophysiology taught him about brain reflexes and the role the brain plays in creating muscular patterns of contraction. Hanna wrote six books, including *The Body of Life* (1980) and *Somatics: Reawakening the Mind's Control of Movement, Flexibility, and Health* (1988). In 1975, he founded the Novato Institute for Somatic Research and Training in Novato, California. He proved through his clinical work that many conditions deemed by doctors to be structural and pathological in nature are, by contrast, functional in nature. Once our sensory motor system improves, our musculoskeletal structure and overall health improve as well.

This book will help you utilize the techniques and methods of Hanna Somatic Education to regain a sense of awareness of and control over your body—a sense that you may not have had for decades. You will learn a simple series of movements that, when done regularly, can bring about more efficient, coordinated, and pain-free physical functioning. My hope is that you will begin to understand that the "mystery" of muscular pain is, in most cases, not all that mysterious. You will begin to experience the ways in which your movement and movement habits affect your entire body.

Regardless of age, muscles can become tight and inflexible, and stop us from living a full, exciting, and active life. For those living with chronic muscular discomfort—and in many cases, chronic pain—navigating this territory can be frustrating and discouraging. I know this from personal experience.

As a former professional dancer who has spent her entire career advising, teaching, and actively working with the body as a performer, dance educator, choreographer, massage therapist, and Hanna Somatic Educator, I am aware of at least ten different methods of pain relief "therapy," some of which work and most of which do not. As one who suffered several repetitive stress and overuse injuries during my dance career—including five knee surgeries and one foot surgery—I, too, spent years looking for just the thing that would get me out of pain and *keep* me out of pain. At the very least, I was looking for someone to give me some solid information that could explain why I—a bodyworker and someone who had spent her entire life working with movement—was in chronic pain in the first place. After all, I was a dancer with solid "core" strength, control of my body, and an extensive knowledge of anatomy, physiology, and movement. I worked out five times a week and could kick my leg right up to my nose. Flexibility was never an issue. During the summers, I climbed mountains, and when my children were young, I could carry a baby in one arm and a stroller and groceries in the other arm without a problem. I was very strong. I had also had ten years of rigorous dance training at some of the premier dance schools in the world. All that knowledge and experience, however, didn't keep me from being in discomfort and/or pain starting from the time I was forty-two years old, with the same problems cropping up time and again. What was it that I was missing? What was it that I hadn't learned? Was I simply getting old and falling apart, a victim of the many injuries I'd had? After all, as one tends to hear when one hits thirty-five, "I wasn't getting any younger!" Was aging really as bad as this? No, that thinking was intrinsically faulty. It was much simpler than that.

When I first began to experience chronic pain, I was working at a chiropractic office. I'd been a massage therapist for fifteen years and maintained a busy practice with happy, loyal clients. I began to notice a trend: many of these clients would visit their chiropractor once or twice a week, come in for their massage, and need to come back and start all over again the next week. It didn't seem right. How could we have survived as a species this long without weekly massages and chiropractic adjustments? It occurred to me that these clients must be *doing* something with their bodies that caused them to regress each week. Our musculoskeletal structure can't be so weak that we need someone to put it back into place for us every seven days. It just didn't add up.

Somatic Education

In 1976, Thomas Hanna coined the term "somatics" to refer to the discipline of movement reeducation—or somatic education—which seeks to foster internal awareness of one's body. To experience something somatically is to experience it in your body: i.e., to be aware of your own bodily sensations and movement from within. Somatic perception is, quite literally, your first-person experience of what it's like to be in your body. Hanna noted that this kind of experience is distinctly different from experiencing your own body from the point of view of another person, such as a doctor, chiropractor, or massage therapist. Early pioneers in the field of somatic education include F. M. Alexander, Gerda Alexander, Elsa Gindler, and Moshe Feldenkrais. Yoga and tai chi can also be considered forms of somatic education. All these disciplines foster a deep sense of internal awareness and an ability to control one's body in space. However, it is Thomas Hanna's discovery of sensory motor amnesia, and his understanding of the reflex patterns our bodies create in response to stress, that distinguish Hanna Somatic Education from all other modalities past and present. It stands alone in its rapid and long-term effectiveness in teaching people to reverse some of the most mysterious (and supposedly structural) conditions responsible for chronic and often debilitating pain: sciatica, scoliosis, chronic back pain, herniated disks, and poor posture, to name a few.

Hanna began his 1988 book, *Somatics*, by relating the ancient riddle of the Sphinx: "What has one voice and yet becomes four-footed and two-footed and three-footed?" According to Greek mythology, Oedipus supplied the answer: the human being. We crawl on all fours in infancy, walk on two legs in adulthood, and then use a cane for support in our old age. Hanna's breakthrough book posed the question of why medical science can protect us from diseases and disorders, extending our lives into our eighties and nineties, but can't seem to explain why we develop muscle tension, stiffness, pain, and inflexibility as we age. Hanna debunked the myth of aging with his discovery of sensory motor amnesia, and used hands-on sessions and somatic exercises to teach those suffering from chronic pain to regain conscious control over and awareness of their own muscles. He advocated independence from the myriad health practitioners whom so many of us rely upon to "fix" us. He exhorted us to improve the function of our sensory motor system in order to regain sensation of and control over our own movements.

Sensory Motor Amnesia

Sensory motor amnesia occurs when your muscles are so tight that they simply won't relax. They are "on" twenty-four hours a day. Even when you're hanging out, enjoying yourself, relaxing, or doing nothing—those shoulders, that hip, that back just won't relax. When massage, chiropractic, heat, cold, stretching, physical therapy, or just about anything else won't relax the muscles for the long term, you probably have sensory motor amnesia.

What it took me a long time to realize, despite all my knowledge about fitness, movement, and bodywork, is that the brain and nervous system control the muscles. Within that connection between the brain and muscles (the sensory motor system), things can become "stuck," due to the brain's response to stress and its constant command to the muscles to tighten. When I learned that the only thing that can permanently change a muscle's tone is *engaging one's brain through movement*—well, I was almost embarrassed by the simplicity of it. Despite all my education, no one had included this bit of specific information in the curriculum. This was indeed the "missing link" for which I had been looking. Within a very short period of time, after having learned the basic concepts and the essential somatic movements in this book, I was able to move without the chronic hip pain that had sidelined me on and off for months. Finally, I was able to move with an ease I hadn't felt in years. Best of all, I was *aware* of and able to *feel* exactly what I had been doing with my body—the very habits that caused the problem in the first place!

Stress is an unavoidable aspect of life. Hanna discovered that it isn't the stress itself that causes muscular problems; rather, the way in which we *reflexively react* to stress over and over and over again throughout our lives determines whether or not we will develop SMA. Simply put, when we get stuck in our stress, then we are in trouble.

What Hanna observed over the course of twenty years of clinical practice was that when muscles become habitually and involuntarily contracted due to real-life stresses such as accidents, injuries, surgeries, major illnesses, repetitive movements, and even emotional situations, not only do those muscles lose their ability to relax, but the brain actually loses sensation of the muscles and forgets how to release them! The end result is tight, sore muscles, joint stiffness, a loss of smooth, controlled movement, and chronic pain. Hanna also observed that during the course of our lives our sensory motor system responds by contracting our muscles in very specific patterns. This can occur at any age. For example:

You're a sixteen-year-old and every day you carry thirty pounds of books on your back, rushing to school, body bent forward. You spend four hours hunched over your computer, doing your homework, then communicating online with your friends. Your mom keeps telling you to stand up straight: you try, but you just can't keep your chest open and your shoulders relaxed. You wind up with stooped shoulders and a painful neck and upper back at a very young age.

You are a young man in your mid-twenties, toned and muscular. You're on the basketball court playing a fast-paced pickup game when your shot is blocked and somehow you fall, landing hard on your right hip. You get up, limp off the court (or maybe you even continue to play), are sore for a couple of days, then feel okay. Every once in a while, that side of your body feels tight. A year later, the knee on the opposite side of your body begins to hurt, even though you never injured your knee. Your hip joint has become extremely tight and you didn't even notice it.

You're a stay-at-home mother of three young children. You always have at least one child on your hip while you go about your daily routine. You have chronic back spasms, but only on one side of your back and buttocks. You find time to take a yoga class, but always come away feeling as if that one spot in your back won't release. Your doctor diagnoses you with sciatica. He says that your skeletal structure has problems.

You're eleven years old, and one day while you're in school a practical joker pulls the chair out from under you. You land hard on your tailbone. You walk slightly bent over from the pain, protecting one side of your body. It happens again a couple of months later. For days afterward, you walk at a slight angle, protecting that painful lower back and pelvis. You sit with most of your weight on one buttock to protect against discomfort. Then at fourteen, you go through a growth spurt—four inches in one summer—and the pediatrician suddenly diagnoses you with scoliosis. One side of your waist muscles has become so tight that it has actually pulled the spine into a curve.

You're seventy years old. You've had a busy life, were never particularly athletic, but you walked everywhere. In the past few years, your daily routine went by the wayside as you took care of your ailing husband, spending hours in the car or in a doctor's office, sitting. You also put on a lot of weight due to your lack of exercise. Now you have trouble walking without pain in your knees. You're told you have arthritis. You feel as if your joints are falling apart.

Every one of these scenarios describes a client of mine. Every one of them had sensory motor amnesia. And every one of them learned how to reverse their SMA so they could get back to a their normal lives without chronic muscular pain. Their problems weren't a result of structural abnormalities. They were issues of sensory motor functioning. These people simply had tight muscles that wouldn't relax. By learning how to use their bodies differently, they were able to positively affect their internal structures and reverse their pain.

The Role of the Brain

To use an analogy familiar to today's computer generation, your brain is the "hard drive" that controls your entire muscular system. When it gets stuck in a feedback loop, then it forgets how to consciously control your muscles and coordinate movement. This is how SMA occurs.

Muscles never move unless the brain gives them a signal to move. It's that simple. If your muscles keep getting the signal to contract—as they do when you tighten and raise your shoulders while you're stuck in traffic or while you answer e-mails at work—they will remain in that position unless you intentionally relax them. Even if they don't remain in an actively contracted position, you will at the very least develop an exaggerated level of muscular tension in your shoulders. Why is this? Because there are two very distinct parts of the brain that have to do with muscle movement: the motor cortex and the subcortex.

The cortex is, for simplicity's sake, the motor of your brain. It receives information from your muscles and tells you how to move. Think back to when you learned how to ride a bicycle. You said to yourself, "Okay, first I get the bike going, then I pick up one foot, now the other, and now I need to balance" . . . and you invariably didn't stay up for long. But after doing it again and again and adjusting your weight and your timing, you finally mastered the skill.

Now here's why—as the saying goes—you never forget how to ride that bicycle once you've learned it: the subcortex. The subcortex is the part of your brain responsible for involuntary movement—that is to say, movement that is already learned and mastered, like eating, writing, throwing a ball, etc.

Let's get back to those tight shoulders: your brain has responded to the stress of the traffic jam by telling your shoulders to tighten and hunch so habitually and consistently that now the shoulders never forget how to sit tighter and higher than is actually comfortable—just as a person never forgets how to ride a bicycle. You don't even have to be in traffic anymore for those shoulders to be tight.

In another example, anyone who sits at a computer and has become completely absorbed by what's on the screen knows how easy it is to slump and get comfortable as you type on the keyboard or surf the Internet. It's no wonder that incidents of carpal tunnel syndrome and neck and shoulder problems are on the rise.

Remember that the brain teaches the muscles to move our bodies in the most efficient manner possible. If you sit for hours with your elbows bent, wrists immobile, and fingers typing away, the brain will teach the arm muscles to hold themselves tighter than usual so that they remain steady, and the neck muscles will hold your head right where it needs to be in order to read what's on the screen. If you are working on a laptop, that downward tilt of your head can result in chronic neck tension.

If your workstation isn't set up ergonomically, your brain will adjust so that your body becomes accustomed to the setup. Eventually this learned posture can lead to tension headaches, TMJ disorder, carpal tunnel syndrome, and neck and shoulder problems.

Let's recap:

Traffic jam: motor cortex of the brain says, "Tighten shoulders." (Or "Tighten neck" or "Tighten arms.") This happens again and again and again.

Subcortex finally says, "I got it; I've learned it. Go on to something else," and takes over the automatic function of tightening the muscles.

Motor cortex goes on to learn something else.

You have effectively set your muscles on cruise control, just as you would set your car.

This is sensory motor amnesia.

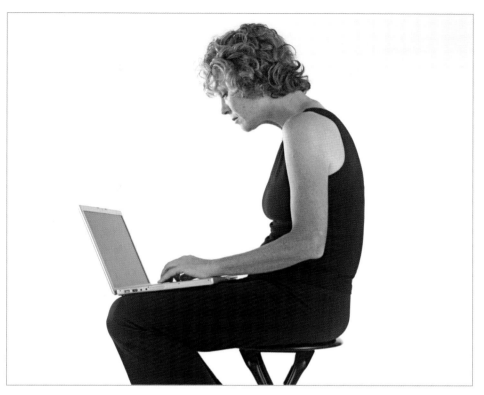

If you are working on a laptop, that downward tilt of the head can result in chronic neck tension.

Is It All in Your Head?

I often have clients ask me, "Do you think my pain is psychosomatic?" My answer is always a firm yes, but I don't say it in an accusatory way. If you take the word "psychosomatic" apart, you have "psycho," meaning mind, and "somatic," meaning relating to the experience of your body in the first person. The mind and the body are one—inseparable—so it goes without saying that one will affect the other. It doesn't mean that a person is crazy, a hypochondriac, or high-strung.

What most medical practitioners mean when they say "It's all in your head" is that a person is just stressed, angry, anxious, or tightly wound, and could really stand to relax a little or just go on vacation. Or maybe address whatever emotional issue is creating the stress in the first place.

In fact, there is no doubt that one's emotional state affects the state of one's muscular system.

This much has already been proven through medical studies conducted decades ago. Dr. John Sarno, author of the 1984 book *Mind Over Back Pain*, wrote about emotional and psychological factors that can create chronic back pain. He felt that the medical profession was too quick to diagnose a structural problem or pathology before looking at the effect of emotional stress on back pain. All mental or emotional stress has the potential to create muscular tension. Ongoing stress can create chronic stress. Thomas Hanna said that "the prevalence of back pain has everything to do with the kind of lives that we live and the kind of society in which we live." The way in which we approach our lives, mentally and emotionally, does impact our muscular system.

However, there's something that doctors are missing when they ascribe all back pain to purely emotional or psychological factors: even if what is occurring *is* initiated by an emotional issue or psychological stress, *your brain responds* by tightening muscles. If a stress reflex, for example, is ongoing, your muscles habituate to the stress, or, if the stress is sudden and violent (as in an accident), the muscular contraction will become involuntary and therefore "stuck" and "frozen" in order to prevent further injury. Every thought that goes through your brain is responded to *muscularly* in your body, whether it is a thought of joy, excitement (as in the experience of watching a scary movie), anticipation, anxiety, fear, or anger. This is part of the finely tuned workings of the sensory motor system (the system in your brain that controls your body): everything that we feel emotionally, sense in our bodies, or experience in our environment is sent as sensory feedback to the brain. The brain integrates this information, and sends motor (movement) commands in response. If any of these stressful situations is long-term or traumatic enough, sensory motor amnesia will take hold. It is then up to you and your brain to regain sensation and control of your muscles and get back to a state of relaxation.

Even if you talk openly about your stress, and rid yourself of suppressed anger and resentment, you still might be left with residual patterns of muscular pain. Serious pain. And that pain is probably the muscular pain of sensory motor amnesia. For those who are sure that emotional or psychological stress is contributing to their pain, it is a wonderful idea to combine a program of somatic education with some other kind of professional therapy that deals directly with emotional issues. Becoming aware of how you respond reflexively in an emotional sense is very helpful in achieving the goal of self-awareness, self control, and physical independence.

It's tough for those who've "tried everything," as I so often hear—those who, despite their best efforts to meditate, chill out, relax, and the like, can't eliminate their pain. Here's where I can help you. Understanding how sensory motor amnesia occurs—and then practicing the gentle movements and innovative techniques you will learn in this book—will help you to become more self-aware, self-monitoring, and self-correcting. You will begin to notice how you reflexively respond when emotions take over, or when unhappiness, anxiety, or the demands of our twenty-first-century life threaten to overwhelm you. Every day we adapt to a changing world, both physically and emotionally. We jump into action or protect ourselves from upset or injury. And sometimes we get stuck in that state of adaptation. By becoming aware of how you deal with life's stresses on a daily basis, you can learn how not to get stuck in your stress!

The Three Reflexes

Thomas Hanna mapped out three distinct, full-body reflexive patterns that people adopt in response to stress. You may look at one of these and think, "That's me!" All three reflexes are important to be able to intentionally go into and come out of—we want to be able to arch and tighten our backs, round ourselves forward, and bend and twist to the side when we want to. We just don't want to get stuck in any one of these patterns.

Green Light Reflex

This reflex, also called the Landau Reflex, is a "call to action" reflex, invoked when there is a need to respond to ongoing demands or stress. We live in an industrialized society in which we are constantly moving, on the go, and working overtime. Our back muscles are constantly tightening to respond to the need to get things done. Think of how you feel when the phone rings, the alarm clock goes off, or you rush out the door in the morning. The back muscles tighten to move us forward so we can accomplish all that we have on our plates. This reflex first occurs at about five months old, when, as infants, we contract our backs to lift our heads and begin to learn to move forward in the

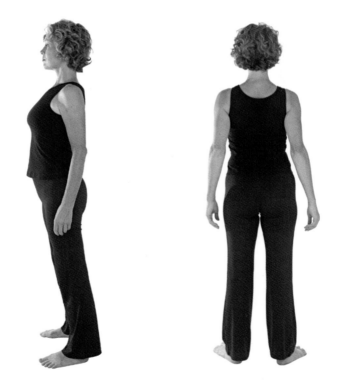

Green Light Reflex: Our back muscles are constantly tightening to respond to the need to get things done.

world. The Green Light Reflex looks like a soldier at attention: the shoulders are pulled back, the neck is tucked in, the pelvis is tilted, and the back muscles are tight and arched. If you can remember back to your childhood when your mother said "Stand up straight!" this was the posture you probably assumed. When habituated, this reflex contributes to a host of conditions like sciatica, lower back pain, neck and shoulder pain, herniated disks, and jaw pain.

Red Light Reflex

Also known as the Startle Reflex, this reflex is a primitive and universal pattern common to all vertebrate animals that occurs in response to anxiety, apprehension,

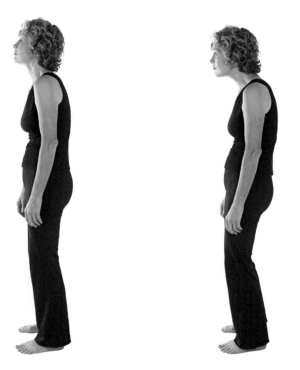

Red Light Reflex: This posture is becoming more common nowadays as a result of long hours slumped over the computer.

fear, or any real or perceived threat. This posture is also becoming more common nowadays as a functional habituation (not an emotional response) to long hours slumped over at the computer.

Think of an animal that senses fear; it instantly crouches down, stops breathing, rounds its back, and curls inward to protect itself until the danger has passed. Humans do the same thing in response to a sudden loud noise or shock, or when we experience fear, anxiety, and depression. Long hours driving or sitting at the computer terminal can also lead to a habituated red light reflex, with hunched and rounded shoulders, tight abdominal muscles and hip flexors, a pelvis that tucks under, and a neck that juts forward. The long-term problems that can result from the red light reflex include shallow breathing, hip and knee problems, neck pain, TMJ disorder, tinnitus, abdominal discomfort, and respiratory problems. Many people assume that this is also the inevitable posture of aging. It is not. It is a learned, habituated posture that can be reversed through careful work with somatic movements.

Trauma Reflex

This reflex occurs in response to accidents or injuries. It is also an avoidance maneuver in which we twist and rotate away in order to escape further injury. When an accident or injury occurs on one side of the body—you slip down a couple of stairs, or sprain your ankle—the waist muscles on the other side tighten in compensation in order to lighten the load on the injured area until everything is healed and back to normal. This occurs unconsciously and instantaneously. And when the waist muscles become tight, the center of the body twists slightly away from the injury. This creates side bending, as well as rotation in the pelvis, shoulders, back, and neck, and can lead to more complicated postural imbalances. If left unchecked, a habituated Trauma Reflex can lead to chronic muscular problems that involve improper leg length, an uneven gait, and tight, painful hips and knees.

Think about it this way: when you have an imbalanced gait due to a habituated twist or a leaning in the center of the body, you are like a car with one flat tire. There is more pressure on one side of your body, and that hip and leg work harder than those on the other side. If you were a car, your tire and axle would eventually wear out. But because you are human, your walking and running are thrown off balance, and one-sided joint problems can develop.

Many doctors are now recognizing scoliosis as a condition that results from trauma, though they don't yet know how to help patients heal it other than with braces and stretching. Somatics can teach even those with scoliosis to make positive changes in their spinal curvature and body alignment.

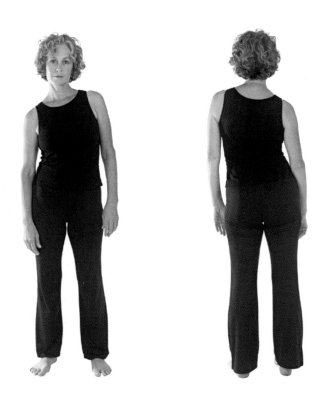

Trauma Reflex: When an accident or injury occurs on one side of the body, the waist muscles on the other side tighten in compensation.

The Myth of Aging

Despite Thomas Hanna's work, the myth of aging is still as alive and well today as it was when *Somatics* was first published in 1988: we simply believe that people reach a certain age and then begin to slow down. Decrepitude sets in, and we cease doing those things that bring us joy: walking, playing tennis, hiking, swimming, dancing, playing with the grandchildren, throwing a ball. Too many in the medical profession still subscribe to this myth, sowing the seeds of despair among their patients.

Ask anyone what "old" looks like in terms of the body: rigid, crunched, hunched over, or clumsy. This perception is caused by the fact that many old people have habitually tight muscles holding them in a stereotypical "old" posture. This description doesn't pertain only to people who are chronologically old: I see these kinds of postures in increasingly younger people. Their rigid, tight muscles and movements are a result of daily functional habits rather than age. Certain specific muscles—in the shoulders, chest, inner thighs, and neck—have responded, via the brain, to everyday stress in such a preprogrammed manner that they can no longer release and relax. In addition, when our muscles become too tight, we also lose our sense of balance. This causes muscles to pull on joints, which causes postural distortions, which causes chronic musculoskeletal pain, leaving people exhausted and depleted, and, in most cases, feeling just plain "old."

In 2006, I took a fall while trying to catch a particularly fast throw in a game of Frisbee. I limped around for a while and pretended to be less hurt than I was. Eventually the pain in my hip went away and I thought I was back to normal. I did begin to notice, however, that I couldn't sit cross-legged quite as well as I'd been able to, and that getting up off the floor caused my left knee to hurt.

I did what I taught others to do, and practiced my somatic movements every day. I tried to figure out why my knee was bothering me. I became an expert of sorts regarding my own knees! After about eight months of annoying pain—which didn't disrupt my life; it was simply bothersome—I decided to go to an orthopedist. The conversation went something like this:

The doctor entered the treatment room, chart in hand. Before examining me, he said, "Ah, knee problems. How old are you?"

ME: Fifty.

DOCTOR: Oh, fifty. Well, you probably have arthritis.

ME: Really? How did that happen?

DOCTOR: That's just what happens at fifty. The joints begin to degenerate. Arthritis develops.

ME: Well, I used to be able to squat down without pain, but now, when I come back up, I have pain.

DOCTOR: Why would you want to squat down anyway? I told you—at your age it's natural for the knee joints to wear down. I'm telling you, you have arthritis. That's just how it is.

Without putting his hands on my knee or checking its range of motion, this doctor decided that I was falling apart due to my age.

An X-ray was taken, then an MRI. I went to a second doctor, who read the MRI and informed me that my pain was the result of a torn meniscus, not arthritis! In fact, he said, "You have not a shred of arthritis in your knee!"

Instinctively, I knew that I didn't have an arthritic condition. Somatically, my intuition was correct! The first orthopedist is still practicing and quite possibly telling his patients that yes, the myth of aging is still intact: your knees naturally fall apart around the age of fifty, and you develop arthritis—so slow down, watch out, be careful. Never mind that in many parts of the world a majority of the population routinely walks miles every day and squats in order to cook, wait for the bus, give birth, or go to the toilet—often at an advanced age.

I see my friends and clients crunching over as they get older and they say, "I'm just getting older. That's how it is. The doctor says that's normal." They take pills. They accept the diagnosis of "age." They believe that to age is to become decrepit, weak, and slow.

Somatics can help you move more intelligently and efficiently as you get older.

We are creatures of adaptation: we adapt to life and all that it brings us. Every day brings change in some area of life, and so every day we change. Our bodies change. We need to know how to adapt to change in a healthy way. Somatics trains your brain to adapt to life's daily changes.

One student asked me, "But you're a somatics teacher. Why would you still need to do the exercises? Why would you still have issues? I mean, aren't you supposed to feel good all the time?"

I feel better than many people my age, but of course I don't feel good all the time. Why? Because every day something occurs that poses a new challenge. That's life. We can't cure all these ailments and aches and be "fixed for life." Life isn't stagnant. Life is movement and change! What we can do is get rid of the dysfunctional patterns of tightness that cause chronic pain, lack of coordination, and inflexibility. For fifteen years I couldn't sit cross-legged or sit on my knees because "I had bad knees," as I would tell people. My hips hurt on and off and I would always have pain in one hip after vigorous exercise. I can now sit cross-legged in a yoga class if I want to. I can sit on my knees for as long as I like without pain or discomfort and I can engage in vigorous exercise without any residual pain. However, I still do my exercises, because I live in our twenty-first-century world: I use a computer, drive a car, and do many repetitive tasks that have a tendency to create sensory motor amnesia. If I do get sore (sitting at the computer being my least favorite activity and one that causes my hips to tighten up), then I know what to do to reverse the situation.

It isn't your age that determines your level of flexibility and well-being, it is what you *bring* to your age that matters. Young children and teenagers who sit at their computers rather than play outside—or who suffer overtraining injuries, ongoing trauma, or illness—are just as likely as adults to suffer from muscular pain. As Thomas Hanna liked to say, "If you're not getting smarter as you get older, you're doing something wrong."

Movement Is Life

There are medical practitioners who will respond to a patient's complaint of muscular pain with exhortations like "Don't exercise," "Be careful," or "Slow down." *Sometimes that advice is appropriate, especially when it comes to a broken bone or a torn muscle.* But at other times, the advice can be detrimental. Surely if exercise keeps causing problems, then maybe you shouldn't be doing it. But it might be *the way in which you're exercising* that's causing the problems.

We humans evolved to move. We learn through movement. Movement is life! Movement isn't something that is done only at the gym. We as a species evolved to walk several miles a day, run, squat, jump, climb trees, and then, when we could afford to (i.e., when we weren't looking for food), rest and lounge. Our bodies are structurally set up for vigorous movement. Our modern industrialized lifestyle, however, has us doing just the opposite: sitting long hours in one position at the computer, driving a car instead of walking, and having machines do the work that once required us to lift, carry, push, and pull. The "slow down, you're not getting any younger" approach to life is an invitation to ill health and decrepitude, not to mention sensory motor amnesia.

As children, most of us are comfortable with movement and, as a result, very aware of our bodies. Then we go to school and the teacher says, "Sit up straight, hands on the desk, eyes straight ahead, don't talk to your neighbor." And we obey, even though it might make us physically uncomfortable. However, as we obey, our brains are teaching us to not pay attention to our internal sensations. We are rewarded for sitting still, not for moving. This is the beginning, for most people, of the loss of our internal awareness of our own bodies—an awareness that is crucial to our well-being.

The most helpful thing to understand in order to keep you moving with flexibility, control, balance, and coordination—well into your old age—is inscribed in the temple of Apollo at Delphi: Know thyself. When you know yourself and pay attention to yourself, you will be well on your way to self-sensing, self-correcting, and ultimately self-healing. Become aware of your body—where it's tight, where it's flexible, where it does or doesn't move. Listen to your common sense and begin to appreciate the beauty and strength of your own body.

Stretching Doesn't Work

All my life I was told to stretch when my muscles felt tight. I could quite easily stretch my leg up to my ear. However, stretching didn't prevent me from getting injured. It is becoming more commonly understood that stretching isn't all it's cracked up to be.

Simply put, stretching doesn't work.

"What?" you exclaim. "But I've been stretching all my life!" Yes, you probably have. You've also probably never felt quite "stretched" and loose afterward, the way you thought you should. You might have even felt that you'd overstretched. And despite all that stretching, you might have injured yourself in the bargain or even strained a muscle or two. Stretching, in many people's experience, implies force. And force rarely gets us where we want to go.

There are many different forms of stretching being taught these days, some of them with names that might make them seem "better" than the standard static stretching we all learned in gym class. We all remember being taught to bend over and reach for our toes. Despite the taut muscles in the backs of our legs screaming out for a reprieve, we were told, "Hold that stretch!" Today, we can learn "dynamic stretching," "resistance stretching," and "active isolated stretching." Some methods are pretty effective, but can be complicated in their instructions and a little vague in their rationales. Other methods require someone to help you. No matter what the name of the technique, when it comes right down to it, stretching is nothing more than pulling.

The basics are these:

Muscles are attached to bones, and bones never move unless the muscles attached to them move them.

Muscles never move unless directed to do so by the brain. The brain controls the entire muscular system. Muscles are controlled by the central nervous system.

> When you stretch, it is safe to assume that there is some level of contraction or tightness in the muscle that you want to loosen.

Now let's think logically: if you have a muscle that is chronically tight, you have a muscle that is holding tension. The involuntary part of the brain is, for some reason, telling that muscle to remain tight. That muscle is no longer under the brain's conscious or voluntary control.

Physically pulling on a muscle with the intention of lengthening it by force or by use of gravity is . . . well . . . just physical. It doesn't require any deliberate action on the part of the brain. Remember—the *brain* controls the muscle.

Pulling a tense muscle past its maximum length invokes a spinal-cord reflex appropriately called the Stretch Reflex. It is a protective reflex that causes an immediate contraction *against* the stretch for the sole purpose of protecting your muscle from overstretching. Your nervous system is trying to help you. It's saying, "Wait! Stop!" When we ignore the Stretch Reflex, what can occur is a further tightening of the muscle, or, in the worst-case scenario, a muscle strain or injury.

So what's missing? What needs to happen is for your *brain to get involved* in teaching the muscle to relax, which will confer greater control and flexibility. Involving the brain will help disrupt the vicious cycle of contraction that keeps our muscles tight.

Start from the very beginning: Unlike animals, who are born with fixed motor patterns, humans learn gradually through movement, a process that takes years. As infants, we are born with certain reflexes (suckling, grasping, flexion), and then, through exploration, sensory feedback, and repetition, we hone useful skills in addition to movement habits that occur in response to the need to adapt. For example, babies learn to feed themselves with utensils by repeatedly lifting the spoon to their mouths until they successfully reach their mouths, a feat that may take them months to achieve. Crawling, walking, running, and reaching are achieved through diligent and persistent exploration, feedback, and repetition. And as we learn motor skills, our brains develop habits that enable us to process additional information and to learn new skills. All these developments occur in the nervous system. This is brain engagement in action.

This exploration-feedback–repetition process shows that the only way the brain learns to control muscle is through movement. This is an important concept to understand when addressing recurring pain or muscular dysfunction. It is crucial to *pay attention* to the way in which we move, or have had to adapt in order to move. This gives us mastery over our bodies and our muscles.

Pandiculation

There *is* an alternative to stretching: waking up your brain and its connection to the muscles—like switching on a light—so that it becomes aware of what's happening in the body. Only then can the brain change what's going on. Simply pulling and stretching the muscle won't work. You must engage the brain in the movement to help you teach the muscle to relax.

So what's the secret to engaging your brain? It's called pandiculation.

Have you ever closely watched a cat or dog get up off the couch, put her paws out, and lengthen herself first on one side of her body and then on the other? It looks like a stretch, but it's not. The animal is pandiculating. She's lengthening entire muscle groups while retaining a bit of tension at the same time. Animals *actively* lengthen from a contraction. They look as if they're doing a full-body yawn. What they do is built-in, automatic, and they do this every time they get up from rest—sometimes up to forty-two times a day! When we lie in bed and yawn, arching our backs and stretching out our legs, that's pandiculation. And it happens at the level of the central nervous system.

Try it for yourself: yawn and pretend that you just woke up. Do you first tighten your arms inward as you yawn, then reach outward slowly? Do you tighten your back at the same time? It feels really good, doesn't it? It should. You are giving your brain lots of feedback about your muscles as you lengthen your muscles from a contraction. Your brain is resetting the muscles' length as the nervous system is waking up the muscles and readying them for action.

Here's another example that might make sense to many of you who are computer-oriented: imagine that your brain is a computer. It controls your muscular system. If your computer is "looping," and no matter what you do it doesn't stop, then you must feed it new information in order to get the program to shut down. Then and only then can you start over.

The only way to achieve that is to make a voluntary, *conscious contraction* that exceeds the force of the contraction you are stuck in, and then the brain will reset the system automatically. It's like hitting Ctrl + Alt + Delete at the brain level. This technique sets Hanna Somatics apart from all other movement programs. It defines the way in which you will work with your body on a daily basis.

A pandiculation is a conscious, voluntary contraction of a muscle—tighter than it already is—followed by a slow, deliberate, and active lengthening of that muscle, followed by a complete relaxation. Just like a yawn. You lengthen the muscle *only to a comfortable length* and not beyond it. That means actively and slowly lengthening to the end of a movement without forcing it. The more you do your somatic movements, the more release and lengthening of the muscle you'll achieve. By paying attention to your own internal sensations and regaining control of your muscles, you are actually giving your brain more feedback and stimulation. You are actively teaching the brain to teach the muscles to relax. This is neuromuscular training at its best. The more sensory stimulation the brain gets, the more information it receives, and the more rapidly it can change what's happening in the body. The brain thrives on stimulation.

Let's review exactly what pandiculation is and how it works.

Every repetitive task we do can result in "frozen," tight muscles. The brain then sets the muscle length to suit whatever condition you have habituated to (slumped posture, tight arms from computer work). Pandiculation—contracting, lengthening, and relaxing—gives the brain a chance to change the muscle length as you contract the muscle past the point of habituation, then lengthen it longer than it was before.

Pandiculation, then, can be defined as a deliberate tightening and lengthening of muscles that therefore resets the brain's motor cortex—the part that teaches us how to do things with our bodies. A pandiculation begins with a voluntary, conscious contraction that exceeds the force of the contraction you are stuck in, thus helping the brain overcome habitual patterns of tightening.

What we do in a pandiculation is threefold:

1. We tighten a specific muscle or muscle group tighter than it already is.

2. We then slowly lengthen and release that muscle or muscles to their full and comfortable length.

3. We then completely relax the muscles.

We *do not* tighten and then immediately relax that muscle completely.

Why? Because this doesn't give the brain the feedback it needs to reset the muscle length. It's important to make the distinction between tightening and relaxing a muscle on the one hand and tightening and *slowly* releasing and lengthening a muscle on the other. Relaxing a muscle doesn't automatically translate into controlling it or increasing its length. You can tighten your shoulders up to your ears, then relax them, but that won't necessarily enable you to notice where your muscle is stuck, or the difference between tight shoulders and relaxed shoulders. When you tighten and then *slowly* release, lengthen, and relax a muscle, you must pay much closer attention to what you're doing. It is in paying close attention with your brain that you successfully rewire those "amnesic" muscles, increasing their range of motion and ability to contract and relax on demand.

A Word About Core Strengthening

"Strengthening the core" is somewhat of a mantra these days. Look at any popular men's health magazine and the first thing you see is a young man with a "six-pack." People think that just because they have tight abdominals they will also be pain-free. Unfortunately, that isn't the case. Athletes, dancers, yoga practitioners, even Pilates instructors aren't immune to muscular pain, despite their core strength. One of the first comments many of my clients make in regard to their back pain is, "I know I should have stronger abdominals . . ."

Yes, conditioned and toned abdominals are important, as is a conditioned and toned body in general. However, what is more important is the *coordination and balance* of those toned muscles rather than how tight they are. Ideally, we should be able to instantly and effortlessly call into action the appropriate muscles needed for a desired task. We should also be able to relax those muscles when they are no longer needed.

The most helpful technique for strengthening your core is full-body exercise. When you use your body as a coordinated system, the movement you are engaging in will dictate whether or not you will need to tighten your abdominals and, if so, how that should be done. Look around at children—running, squatting, bending, climbing, reaching, pulling, and pushing. Not only are their abdominals toned without being rigid—relaxed and ready to be contracted when needed— but their bodies are also able to perform all the normal activities of play. They are, generally speaking, coordinated and agile, able to move on different planes—up, down, front, back, high, and low. Their bodies are healthy and strong because of all the vigorous, full-body movement involved in play—not because they do sit-ups and crunches.

If you want to strengthen your core, you're better off finding a pleasurable full-body activity to participate in—one in which sensory motor and balance skills are tested and honed—than sweating through the repetitive drills that many of us perform on machines at the gym. These drills isolate muscle groups— an approach that not only has no relationship to functional movement in our daily lives, but may also cause muscular tightness that impedes fluid movement.

Make It Fun!

My favorite quote about exercise comes from the book *Play as if Your Life Depends on It,* by Frank Forencich:

Warning: Before beginning a program of physical inactivity, consult your doctor. Sedentary living is abnormal and dangerous to your health.

All the somatic movements you will learn in this book shouldn't take the place of what you enjoy doing. But prepping yourself with somatic movements will *keep* you enjoying whichever physical activity you love to do. Just as a cat or dog pandiculates before getting up from rest, so should we. Then we should get out and move! Our bodies are designed for vigorous movement and our brains are designed to teach us to learn through movement. More and more is being written about the positive affects of vigorous, daily movement on brain plasticity, brain-cell growth, emotional states, learning disabilities, and behavioral problems. The more you move, the smarter you become and the easier it is to focus and concentrate. If you want to be healthy and strong for the long term, you *must move.* There's no avoiding it.

Many of my clients are amazed at how relaxed and aware they feel after doing the somatic movements in this book. Some say that they can't believe it's so easy to feel so good, and they wonder what the gimmick is. There's no gimmick. It's just your brain, your muscles, and a natural sense of satisfaction after learning to do something new and different.

But why are my clients so surprised? Maybe because most of us are taught that in order to learn something or get stronger, you have to "feel the burn," you have to suffer. Sure—if you want to become an elite athlete or dancer, climb Mount Everest, or engage in extreme sports, you will have to endure years of training in which sore muscles are an everyday occurrence. I speak from experience when I say that there can be a certain amount of suffering involved in pushing your body that way. However, as a former dancer, I can also assure you that sensory motor learning—knowing where your body is in space and knowing how to control what you're doing—is the only way to master any activity. If you can feel the relationship between your feet, legs, hips, back, shoulders, and neck, you're on your way to effortless and efficient movement—no matter how old you are.

If you want to build muscles and endurance in order to be able to lift your children, carry your groceries, walk long distances, run, and play just for the fun of it—not to mention age well—suffering and straining past your reasonable limit doesn't need to be a part of it. It's true that you do have to put some effort into it. Becoming strong isn't a pill you can swallow that will cause you to morph magically into Lance Armstrong. It requires consistent effort. However, intelligent, aware control of your muscles is the single most crucial element of any physical activity you participate in. Otherwise, you won't be in control of your own body enough to know when you've gone too far.

Anything worth doing is worth doing effortlessly.   —*Anonymous*

I am often asked for advice about what kind of exercise to do. Many of my clients don't want to return to the repetitive exercises that caused them injury. Some do want to return to their previous activities (yoga, tennis, Pilates, hiking, running), but aren't sure if they're going to get injured again. I tell them that if they do the daily somatics movements and improve awareness of their bodies, they will be more in control of the movements inherent in their activities. The more aware you are, the less likely you will be to get injured or to push yourself beyond what is comfortable. If you do overdo it, you have techniques—the movements—to reset yourself and your muscles.

Many of my clients say that they find exercise to be a tedious, crashing bore. They tell me they go to the gym not because they enjoy it, but because they think they should. Some even have personal trainers, spend vast amounts of money on them, and dread the workout. Why is this? Maybe it's because we've forgotten the most important rule about exercise: it should be pleasurable!

There's a reason for this: if something is pleasurable, we are more likely to want to repeat it. If it is not pleasurable, we will make a million excuses for avoiding it. Many of us know how laborious it can be to go to the gym, count our repetitions, walk on the treadmill, and do what it is we think we *should* do as opposed to what it is we *enjoy* doing.

At this point, it is important to make the distinction between exercise and movement. Exercise is a repetitive activity, the goal of which is to achieve a certain level of strength and proficiency. Movement is a fluid activity that plays a functional role in daily life. A movement-filled life is one in which exercise is made obsolete.

I find it refreshing when I meet someone who says, "I love being outside, so I just walk." People like this often seem apologetic, but I assure them they're on the right track—especially if walking is what they love to do and it keeps them moving! If you love going to the gym, keep going. If you don't, no worries—there are plenty of enjoyable alternatives, such as the ones I've listed below. You may also refer to the resources section in the back of the book for more exercise and fitness ideas.

Walking

Dr. Andrew Weil, in his book *Spontaneous Healing*, says that walking is the "exercise" practiced by most of the world on a daily basis because it is most people's primary form of transportation. He adds that walking not only provides aerobic activity, but also helps on a proprioceptive and neuromuscular level as well. Walking is a cross-patterned movement—something it has in common with the movements in this book—because, as we walk, we swing our arms in opposition to the direction in which our legs and feet are moving. Cross-patterning is important for brain development (think of babies crawling), and helps the central nervous system learn to coordinate movement.

Walking was the most important adaptation and survival mechanism in human evolution. We evolved to walk long distances, with arms and shoulders that counterbalance our legs and hips. It was not uncommon for hunter-gatherers to walk up to eight miles a day in order to find food. Still, today, in many developing countries people will walk between five and ten miles a day just to get to and from work. Walking, hiking, and moving outdoors stimulates the brain and calms the mind. Explore your environment, notice your surroundings, fill your lungs with air, and be aware of your stride. So find a destination—be it the grocery store, your local park, or a nearby mountain—and start walking!

Dancing

Dancing, like play, has been around a long time, and is considered one of the most enduring forms of tribal worship. In many cultures around the world, dancing is what people do when they gather together. Young and old, fat and thin will dance as a joyous way of socializing. You don't have to be trained to dance! It has the added benefit of helping to improve your sense of balance, which often diminishes as we age. In addition to being one of the most pleasurable and social pastimes there is, dancing also incorporates brain-to-muscle learning (sensory motor learning), and enhances proprioception and coordination. I have been known to tell my clients to go home, put on their favorite music, and dance.

Play

I think it's safe to say that the oldest form of exercise around is play. Yes, play. Think about it: young animals play, children play, and babies play. They can do it for hours on end with only brief interruptions for rest. Play is both a physical and social experience. When children play, they change their games, make up new rules, start and stop, but never seem to get tired. They learn about the world through play. Without play, kids suffer all kinds of ills. Play is "exercise" for kids. Play-based fitness will tone and strengthen you, and help to improve coordination and balance—while you laugh and have fun—as no other exercise can.

Frank Forencich, the author of *Play as if Your Life Depends on It*, recommends that we inject some aspects of play into our walking or running routines. For example, we can mix fast and slow movements: walk, then sprint, jump, or hop; walk, skip, then walk again. Put on your headphones or earbuds, choose some lively tunes, and dance down the street (I've done this—no joke). Your neighbors might think you've lost your mind, but you'll be having a great time! Change the terrain and walk over rocks and down hills. This will not only improve your sensory awareness, balance, and proprioception, but it will force you to engage your core muscles for good balance.

Many playful activities—such as throwing and catching a ball with a partner, climbing a wall (many towns now have places to safely learn to do this), riding a bicycle, and, of course, dancing—enable us to engage in "functional fitness," defined as exercise that involves patterns of movement you use on a daily basis.

So let's play a game. Close your eyes and imagine yourself as a child—outside in your backyard, a local park, the school playground, or wherever you used to play. Which games were your favorites? Choose one and start playing it in your imagination. Feel your heart, your breathing; feel how your sense of time disappears and your imagination soars. Are you with friends or alone? What are you doing? Jumping rope? Playing freeze tag? Climbing on the monkey bars? Playing manhunt in the dark? Sneaking through the grass barefoot, like a tracker? Feel your arms, legs, feet, all moving together. Bring your game to a close as you lie on the ground, exhausted and exhilarated. Now open your eyes. How do you feel? What did you notice about your body? Play does a body good, doesn't it?

Hula-Hooping

Who remembers Hula-Hoops? Hooping, as it is now called, is making a comeback. It is very somatic. It requires you to become aware of the movement in the center of your body as you gently undulate from front to back and side to side to keep the hoop twirling. It works the abdominal muscles, hips, and back, and improves coordination—all while you have a blast! I discovered that although it *looks* difficult, Hula-Hooping relies on a simple undulating rhythm that comes from the center of the body; your movement becomes smoother and more controlled as you respond to the feedback of the hoop around your waist. This can increase brain plasticity, allowing us to stay flexible and healthy. Forget crunches and sit-ups—try hooping for twenty minutes every day (the time will absolutely fly by!) and you'll feel tall, strong, and centered.

Swimming

Swimming is a low-impact, full-body activity that everyone can enjoy. It's a great way to learn to sense imbalances in your movement (notice which arm reaches farther as you do the crawl stroke) and begin to change them. It's easy on the joints and great for developing cardiovascular stamina and muscle strength.

Going Barefoot

The notion of taking off our shoes and going barefoot is gaining popularity. Thanks, in part, to the success of the book *Born to Run* by Christopher McDougall, more and more people are beginning to shed their shoes and feel their feet. McDougall chronicles his experiences running with the greatest distance runners in the world—the Tarahumara Indians of Mexico, who run between fifty and one hundred miles at a go—all while wearing thin, homemade huaraches on their feet.

One of the first things I ask my clients who have foot, knee, or hip problems is, "Do you ever walk barefoot?" I've had responses that vary from "I never go barefoot. It gives me the creeps!" and "Really? Won't I hurt myself?" to "I've always loved going barefoot, but I've been told not to." I remind my clients that the twenty muscles of our feet are no different from any other muscles in our bodies. If you lose sensation, function, and control of your feet, you are at greater risk of developing a problem elsewhere in your body.

Our feet, hands, and mouths are among the body's most important sensory organs. Infants play with their feet, which enriches the brain's awareness of the body. Toddlers walk barefoot, using all the muscles of their feet to help balance themselves. As we get older, we encase our feet in shoes, because we've been told that we need the support. We're told that flat feet, sore feet, and pronated feet need arch supports. I know a pediatrician, now in his eighties, who said that when he was in medical school, they were taught that muscle function and flexibility of the feet had more to do with foot pain than anything else. If children retain the flexibility in their feet, even the presence of common minor foot problems—flat feet, for instance—will likely never bother them.

If we constantly wear shoes, we can't feel the ground. If we can't *sense* our feet, we lose the ability to use the muscles in them. Scott McCredie, in his book, *Balance*, writes that the loss of awareness and control of one's feet, and the wearing of cushioned shoes, is implicated in the increasing number of falls suffered by senior citizens. Any movement executed in gravity requires intelligent use and coordination of the feet. Allow them to get lazy, and they'll have trouble stabilizing us, flexing, extending, inverting, and everting. Balance needs to be improved as we age, and balancing exercises are now a part of many movement routines for seniors. However, without the ability to feel and move your foot muscles, balancing exercises will have little effect. Learning to use your feet will help you stay more in control of your movement so you don't lose your balance. Remember the song "Dem Bones"? "The knee bone connected to the thigh bone" Well, it's true.

Think of ballet dancers who perform the most intricate movements, often at lightning speed. They wear thin slippers. Can you imagine how a ballerina might move while wearing sneakers? Dancers and athletes use the muscles of the feet to give them more spring as they jump and more cushioning as they regulate their landings.

Mick Dodge—known as the Barefoot Sensei—once asked the question, "What's the first thing that happens when you take your shoes off?" The answer: "You start paying attention." And paying attention to your entire body and its movement is what this book is about.

So take off your shoes and walk. Be mindful, go slowly, and feel your feet. Then notice what the rest of your body does. I think you'll find it addictive.

As You Begin

If you have a brain and a body, this book is for you. If you are active, inactive, recovering from an injury, feeling "old," dealing with an ongoing condition, feel as if you've forgotten how to move, or simply want to maintain awareness and flexibility as you age, then this book will benefit you. It teaches internal awareness, something that every one of us is at risk of losing as we age.

As we go through life, we continue to learn and grow. We develop habits, physically and emotionally, in order to adapt to our circumstances. The endocrinologist Hans Selye (1907–1982) identified what he called the General Adaptation Syndrome in 1936. In his book *The Stress of Life*, he stated, "All disease is disease of adaptation," and asserted that whether stress is positive (eustress) or negative (distress), it has a major impact on health. He wrote that our attitudes, sense of self-responsibility, and choices in dealing with stress—an awareness that comes from the inside out—can go a long way toward reducing any negative impact stress might have. This applies as surely to how we adapt to the need to sit over the computer for long hours or hold a baby on our hip as it does to how we will to ride a bicycle. And because many unhealthful physical habits come about through learned behavior, we can, when made aware of them, go about unlearning them. Sensory motor amnesia is reversible. In learning the movements and concept in this book, you will be encouraging the brain to remember, in some cases, complex movements that at the outset might seem impossible. That's okay. With patience and persistence, you'll soon find yourself quite comfortable with a new way of moving.

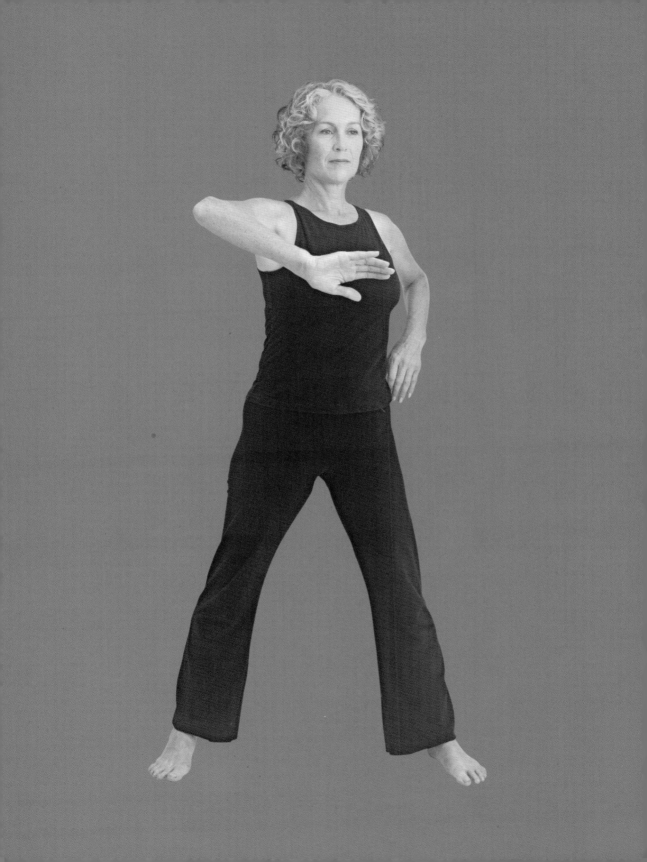

PART II

The Movements

How to Use This Book

Regaining movement where muscles were once tight and sore is a process of remembering. I guarantee that there is no one in the world who knows how your body functions—or cares how your body functions—more than you. Remember what "soma" means—the living body in the first person. You are the only one living in your body, so you are, ultimately, the expert!

I have ordered the movements in a specific way to enable you to release and relax your muscles from the inside out, thereby allowing you to derive the most lasting benefit from your practice sessions. Randomly choosing a few movements that you like is fine, but if you *really* want to become the master of your body, it's best to begin with those that methodically wake up the body, slowly but surely.

By doing the movements in the order in which they appear, you will experience a slow, progressive awakening of the muscles—not only in the center of your body, but also in the appendages. By releasing the back muscles and the abdominals first, it will be easier to go on to the movements for the waist and hips. Those movements will in turn prepare you for slightly more complicated movements. As you do them, your brain is resetting itself, establishing a new, heightened sensory awareness, more finely tuned motor control, and better physical coordination.

From Core to Periphery

In Hanna Somatics, we focus on releasing, relaxing, and regaining control in the center of the body first, and then in the periphery of the body. After all, what goes on in the center of your body affects what goes on in the periphery! For example, if a client comes to me with pain in his foot or knee, I first observe the way in which he walks and stands, rather than looking at the foot or knee as separate from the rest of the body, as many specialists do. Perhaps when he stands, he's putting more weight on one foot. That would surely cause some discomfort over time. Maybe one hip isn't moving as much as the other hip when he walks. Maybe his tight back muscles are pitching him forward in his stride, which causes him to come down roughly on his heel.

Here's another example: imagine that you're wearing a corset. Now imagine reaching up high for something on the top shelf of your kitchen cabinet. How far could you actually reach? Now imagine taking that corset off and reaching way up high, letting your entire body lengthen as you do. I'll bet you can anticipate how much easier it would be. It's okay to have a nice toned core—and it's crucial to have abdominal support—but it will not serve you in the long run to have a six-pack if you cannot voluntarily release and relax those tight muscles in order to twist, turn, reach, and bend.

Overly tight abdominal muscles also make deep, full breathing difficult. When the center of the body can't relax, it's more difficult for the ribs to expand and the lungs to draw in a deep breath. Babies, as you may have noticed, breathe from their bellies. Unless they are in distress, you will never see babies breathing shallowly from their upper chests or shoulders. They will always breathe deeply from the bottoms of their lungs. Their bellies rise and fall with each breath.

Then babies learn to get up and walk. What a feat that is! They have to coordinate all those trunk muscles to balance themselves, but they do it. Then they grow older and continue running, rolling, reaching, jumping, squatting, and doing all the things that kids do. All these natural activities tone the core muscles at the center of their bodies, which coordinate together in a balanced manner. Children without back pain don't sit at computers all day, drive cars that get stuck in traffic jams, or worry about bills. But the more time they spend hunched over electronic toys, cell phones, and video games, the more they lose control and awareness of the core muscles of their bodies. Some of them exhibit the same stress-related muscular problems found in many thirty- and forty-year-olds. The good news is that all the movements of childhood are movements that we adults can remember if we simply take the time to reacquaint ourselves with our own bodies.

Aging occurs—but life is movement, whether it be breathing or dancing! So let's get started!

The Gift of Awareness

The single most important gift that you will give to yourself by doing these somatic movements every day is one of awareness. If you don't want to spend the rest of your life going to myriad practitioners every time you have an ache or pain, increasing awareness of the way in which you move will help you more than any other single factor. Many people think that back pain, for example, suddenly happens *to* them—that somehow they are unwitting victims. The truth is that everything we do and everything that happens to us is responded to muscularly in the body. Our reactions to stress occur from the inside out. Becoming aware of your habitual response to stress and your movement habits is the first step to reversing muscle pain, poor posture, and limited movement. Consider the following questions:

How do you sit in your car (slumped or with an arched back)?

How do you sit at your computer (slumped, with an arched back, or slightly angled, with your monitor at one angle and your body at another)?

How do you walk (with your heel striking, bouncing on the balls of your feet, smoothly, or swaying from side to side like Frankenstein)?

What do your footsteps sound like? Do you clomp heavily? Do you shuffle your feet?

How much movement do you have in your arms when you walk? Do they move easily or stiffly?

How do you stand (always on the same foot, or with your weight on both feet)?

How do you reach, bend down, or carry things?

How do you respond to long hours at the computer? Do you slouch, sit up ramrod straight, arch your back and tilt your pelvis forward, or jut your neck out?

It is in the noticing of your own patterns that you can become more self-monitoring and self-correcting. Sometimes it's as simple as noticing how you arch your lower back when you *think* you are sitting up "straight."

How to Get the Most Out of the Movements

The slower you go, the more your brain teaches your body.

—*Thomas Hanna*

Anyone who has ever played the piano, rehearsed a difficult dance step, perfected his golf swing, or learned to knit knows that in the beginning you must move slowly in order to sense, coordinate, and control your movements. You must be aware of what your hands, feet, arms, torso, and fingers are doing. Then, when you are practiced in your movements, you can speed things up. That's when your skills will become second nature. Remembering how to move muscles that have been guarding due to an accident or trauma, or have simply been tight and sore for a long time requires that you apply the same principle—proceed slowly at first.

Here are some other tips to help you get started:

Remember that many of the movements are pandiculations. I frequently ask my clients to imagine that they're moving as if they are just waking up in the morning—almost as if they were yawning.

Move slowly, gently, and with awareness.

Don't attack the movements as though they're something to be gotten out of the way, or quotas to be achieved at the gym. Enjoy them—they're pleasurable, not taxing.

Be consistent with your practice. You will get longer-lasting results if you remember that all learning, whether in sports, dance, or chess, requires persistence.

Be patient with yourself, and maintain a positive attitude. Rome wasn't built in a day.

Wear loose, comfortable clothing.

Make sure that you have a quiet place in which to do your movements, as any distraction—be it music, the cat, or the TV—can interfere with your concentration. Here is a case where the ability to multitask is a liability.

It is best to do your movements on a rug or yoga mat in order to have a firm support for your body. If you are infirm or incapable of getting down on the floor, you can do your movements in bed. However, the results will probably not be as good as if you were to do them on the floor.

These exercises should not be painful! If you experience some mild pain when contracting a muscle, simply contract that muscles *only as far and as much as is comfortable*. Go "up to the edge" of that discomfort, and relax out of it. There's no sense in trying to move through pain. If a muscle is sore when you're moving, and that soreness, doesn't subside after a couple of days of doing the movements, then stop. Forcing movement can not only cause injury, but can also distract the brain from sensory awareness and feedback.

Remember to *completely* relax after each repetition. Otherwise, you'll still retain a small amount of muscle tension. Try not to be ready and primed for the next repetition. When you completely relax, you're giving your brain the opportunity to absorb both the sensory feedback from the muscles and the sensation of relaxation.

A very small percentage of people may become a little bit sore for about twenty-four hours after beginning these movements. The soreness should go away after a day or so. This can occur because you're "waking up" muscles that have been contracted for a long time. A muscle that has been contracted or in spasm for a long time will often be sore once it is relaxed.

Sensory motor amnesia often shows up as jerky, shaky movements, or areas of movement that just aren't as smooth as you'd like them to be—like a skip in a vinyl record album. When you sense that shaky movement, or anything in that range of motion that doesn't feel under your control, *slow down*. Go back, recontract that tight muscle slightly, then slowly release out of it and see if you can make the movement smooth. It's always best to do what your brain already knows how to do (which is to hold the muscle tightly), and then slowly and gently nudge the muscle into its new range. You're using intelligent movement to create a change in the muscle, rather than force.

Quality of movement is important. Try to perform the movements slowly and smoothly.

People often like to find a "trick" to release one joint or muscle—their tight hip, for instance. But before you jump ahead to a movement intended to relax that tight hip, don't forget to first do some basic movements to relax the back, front, and waist muscles. Then go on and target that hip. Addressing postural abnormalities or recurring trouble spots in the one part of the body works best when you address SMA in the entire body. Just as a ballet dancer begins her routine with gentle demi-pliés before going into leaps and turns, so should you remember to pay attention to the basics first.

You'll soon find that fifteen minutes of performing the somatic movements in this book—which are based on the work of Thomas Hanna and other practitioners, such as Moshe Feldenkrais, Marilyn Warnock, and Frank Forencich—will prepare you beautifully for whatever activity you enjoy doing, be it yoga, running, or walking. All the movements are safe, natural, and common to the human movement "vocabulary." After a few days of practicing them, you may even notice that your movement becomes easier and more efficient—that you're no longer having to work so hard to move. This is what we're looking for—effortless, easy movement. Now go and have fun!

1

Sensing

To become aware of your body, you must first pay attention to what your brain can and cannot sense. Are you aware of where your feet are lying when you're on your back? Where is your lower back on the floor? How are your hands lying? These are the simple, basic beginnings of somatic movement. Becoming aware of how your body is positioned enables you to identify which of your muscles are contracted.

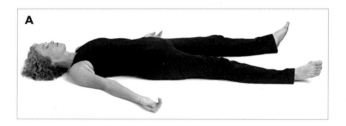

A. Lie on your back with your legs comfortably extended on the floor and your arms at about a 45-degree angle away from your body.

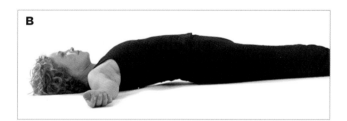

B. Sense your lower back. Is it arched up off of the floor, as in the photo, or is it lying comfortably and evenly on the floor?

How are your feet lying? Are they flopped out equally, or is one foot pointing toward the ceiling while the other is comfortably flopped out? Where on the heels do you feel the weight of your body?

Sense the length of your neck. Is it relaxed and long or is it arched and curved? Is your head touching the floor in the middle of your head or more toward the upper part of your head?

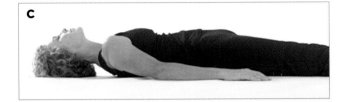

C. Sense what your shoulders feel like. Are they rounded up off the floor or are they comfortably relaxed? Notice any tightness through your chest. Try to sense whether you have rounded shoulders, as in the photo.

NOTICE AND SENSE

Breathe deeply and notice how your breath feels. Is it easy to take a deep breath? How far does the breath go up into your chest?

Gently roll your head from side to side as if shaking your head "no." What do you feel? Can you feel anything in your shoulders when you do that? Is there any movement there? Is one shoulder tighter than the other?

Finally, sense whether one side of your body feels heavier than the other side. If so, is it the same side as a hip or foot that is less relaxed? If you were lying on the beach, and were magically lifted up off the ground, what would your impression in the sand look like? Would you have a deeper impression on the right or on the left?

2

Arch and Flatten

This movement, in which the entire back of your body moves gently, is aimed at returning control of your back muscles to your brain. You are creating the Green Light Reflex voluntarily, then relaxing out of it. This will improve your ability to intentionally relax your back muscles when they are no longer needed for an activity. You are also regaining an awareness that, when your back tightens, the front of your body wants to simultaneously relax and lengthen.

When you inhale, make sure you're breathing "from the belly." You can even place a hand over your navel and notice how your hand rises with the movement of the belly when you inhale. If you find it difficult to inhale and allow your belly to expand and relax, go slowly and do the best you can.

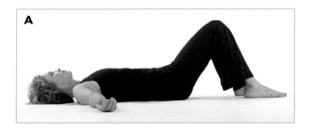

A. Begin with your knees up and your feet planted near your buttocks. Then place your arms at your sides, slightly away from your body. Take several deep breaths into your lower lungs, and allow your abdominals to relax and lengthen. This is called a belly breath, because you allow your belly to inflate like a balloon, instead of sucking it in, as many people do when inhaling. You should be aware of your breathing throughout this movement.

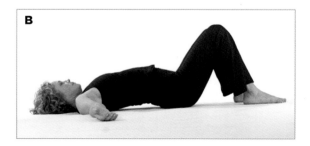

B. Inhale and slowly roll your tailbone down into the floor or mat as you allow your lower back to arch slightly. Arch only to a comfortable height.

When you tilt your pelvis, your lower back muscles are contracted and arched, and your tailbone is rolled down in the direction of your feet. The front of your body is relaxed, lengthened, and open.

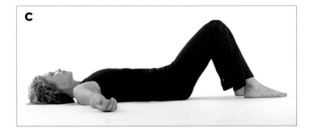

C. Exhale and allow your back to float down to the floor or mat, as your tailbone rolls back to neutral.

Repeat this movement for around a minute, or about 10–15 times.

NOTICE AND SENSE

Sense how your abdominal muscles relax and lengthen as you inhale, and how your back muscles tighten as you arch and roll your tailbone down. Roll your pelvis and arch your back only as far as is comfortable.

Notice that your neck is pulled long as you arch. You're tight in the back and released in the front. As you exhale and relax your back, it lengthens as your pelvis gently rolls back to a neutral position. You are moving all the muscles from your tailbone up to your neck. There is a connection between your neck and tailbone!

Notice also that you are pandiculating the back muscles as you arch and relax. This is like a slow yawn you might indulge in before getting up in the morning.

Allow your back to float down to the floor or mat. Don't deliberately push or tighten it down. I want you to get the feeling of contraction, then active relaxation and lengthening. Make this movement smooth and fluid, like a wave.

3

Arch and Curl

This movement focuses on the abdominal muscles, or flexor muscles, which work together with the back muscles, or extensor muscles. We want the back and abdominal muscles to work together so that one side doesn't dominate the other. When the abdominals are too tight, they can restrict breathing and pull the chest wall down, which can also create a co-contraction in the back muscles. This movement will help you avoid that pattern and regain awareness and control of your abdominal muscles. Be sure to move slowly. This is not a sit-up! It's a controlled movement of the front and back of the body that, when done slowly, helps to coordinate the back muscles and the abdominals easily and effortlessly.

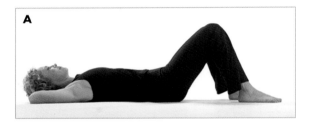

A. Lie on your back with your knees up and your feet planted near your buttocks. Place both hands, with fingers interlaced, behind your head. Rest your elbows on the floor or mat.

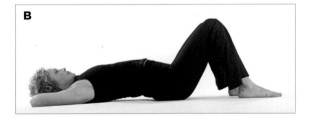

B. Inhale and slowly arch your lower back while you roll gently your tailbone gently down in the direction of your feet. Your back is tight and your front is relaxed and lengthened.

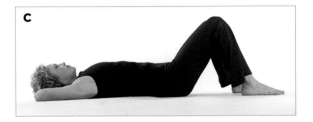

C. Exhale and slowly allow your back to relax down to the floor.

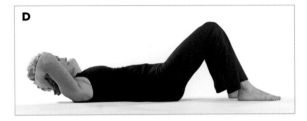

D. When your back is on the floor, flatten it firmly, tuck your chin into your chest, pick your head up with your hands (to protect your neck), and tighten your abdominal muscles as you round up.

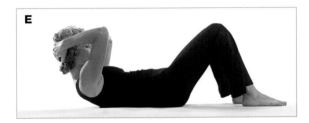

E. Bring your elbows inward toward each other, and point them in the direction of your knees, so as to widen your back. Engage your ribs to tighten the entire abdominal muscle from your pubic bone up into your ribs.

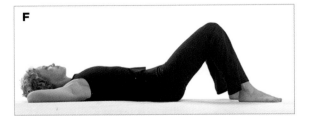

F. Inhale and slowly roll back down to the floor. Be sure to lengthen your abdominals as you come down.

Repeat this movement 4–6 times.

Arch and Curl *(continued)*

NOTICE AND SENSE

Sense how the extensor muscles of your back lengthen from the tailbone up to the base of your skull as you curl yourself up toward your knees. Meanwhile, your abdominals are tight, your ribs are pulled down, your pelvis tilts toward the center, and your back is long.

The *rectus abdominus* muscle extends from the pubic bone up into the ribs. It is a long, wide muscle. Sense how, when this muscle contracts, the ribs are pulled down toward the pelvis, and the pelvis is pulled upward toward the ribs. When you relax back down and lengthen through the front, the ribs gently lift and relax. This will help increase your capacity to breathe.

You don't need to curl up a lot in order to gain awareness of your abdominals. You can simply pick your head up gently, as if you want to look at your belly button. When you sense your abdominals tightening, slowly come back down.

If your neck is bothering you in general, then you might suspect a battle between the muscles in the back and the front of the body—in other words, a battle between the Green Light Reflex, in which the muscles in back are tight, and the Red Light Reflex, in which the muscles in front are tight. Once you gain the ability to consciously contract and release those muscles in concert with each other, you will find your neck feeling better.

4

Back Lift

This movement addresses all the muscles in the back of the body that contract in response to activity and ongoing stress.

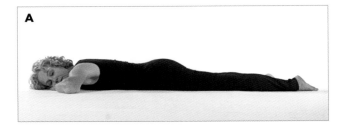

A. Lie on your stomach and place your right cheek down on the back of your left hand with your right arm resting lengthwise alongside your body. Get comfortable, and make sure that your left shoulder is relaxed.

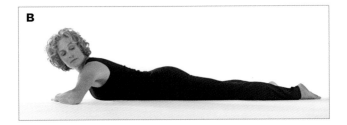

B. Leave your left elbow on the floor and slowly lift your upper body. Sense how far down your back you can feel the contraction. This movement resembles what a baby does when she looks around for the first time, at around five months of age. It's called the Landau Reflex. Your abdominals should be soft as your back contracts to bring you up. Repeat this several times, slowly.

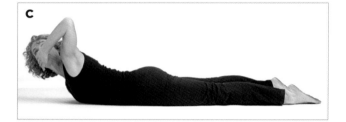

C. Slowly lift your elbow, head, and hand off the floor as if you wanted to look over your left shoulder. Relax your right arm on the floor or mat. Lift only as far as is comfortable. Keep your nose facing your elbow. You may only come up about two inches—that's fine. Sense the contraction in your upper body between your shoulder blades and down into your lower back. You tighten the back of your body while the front of your body lengthens. Slowly come back down to the floor and completely relax.

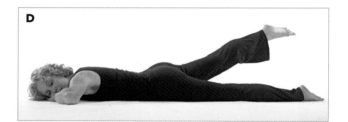

D. Now just lift the right leg. Keep your knee straight. Notice how the opposite shoulder automatically presses down into the floor. The leg and the shoulder work together. Sense the contraction in your lower back muscles as you lift your leg. Bring it down slowly, and feel your lower back muscles lengthen. Completely relax.

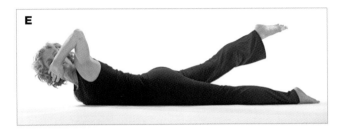

E. Now, with your left hand and cheek "glued" together, inhale, and at the same time slowly lift your head, hand, and elbow while also lifting your right leg up off the mat as far as is comfortable. *Slowly* bring yourself back down to the mat. Control the movement and make it smooth.

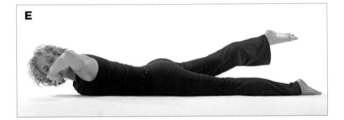

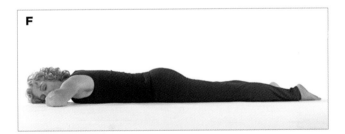

F. *Completely* relax on the mat and sense your back muscles. Remember to completely relax your neck as well.

Repeat this movement 3–4 times on each side.

Back Lift *(continued)*

Variation

If your neck is particularly tight and uncomfortable, this is a nice, easy variation on the above movement.

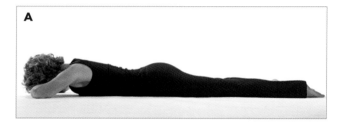

A. Lie with both hands palm down, one on top of the other. Rest your forehead on your hands. This is the position you will return to after each repetition.

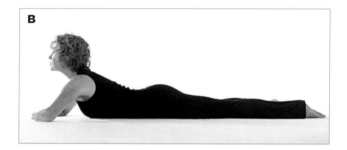

B. As you inhale, slowly tighten your back to lift your head. Feel your belly go down into the floor as your head lifts up. Sense the contraction all the way down your back. Slowly relax your back and bring your head back onto your hands.

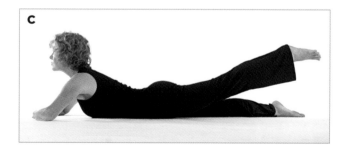

C. Inhale, then lift your head and your right leg simultaneously. Slowly lower both your head and leg, and completely relax. The back lengthens as you bring your head and leg down to neutral.

Repeat with your left leg.

NOTICE AND SENSE

Sense how, when one side of the upper body contracts, the opposite side of the lower body automatically contracts to achieve balance. The shoulder and back muscles of one side and the lower back, gluteus, and hamstring muscles of the other side all contract together to balance your movement. This is natural and involuntary.

Sense how your front lengthens and your back contracts as you do this movement.

You're pandiculating your back muscles by tightening them as you lift up, then actively and slowly lengthening and releasing them as you lower yourself down. Do this as gracefully as you can.

Remember to *completely melt* into the floor or mat, and let your brain absorb the sensation of relaxation of the back muscles.

You're learning to control all the deep muscles of your back in doing this movement.

5

Diagonal Arch and Curl

This movement focuses on the "red light" muscles of the abdominals—the ones that contract in the Red Light Reflex. When you contract your abdominals, you simultaneously lengthen your back muscles. The deeper you drop your back toward the floor while doing this movement, the easier it will be for you to round up toward your knee.

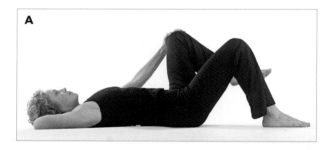

A. Lie on your back with your knees bent and your feet near your buttocks. Put your right hand under your head. Bring your left knee up and grab it with your left hand. Just let it balance over your hip as in the photo.

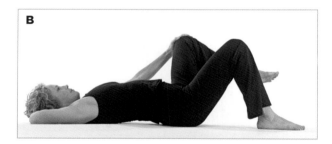

B. Inhale, allowing your back to arch as you roll your tailbone gently down into the floor. Let your knee move a little in order to allow for the arch.

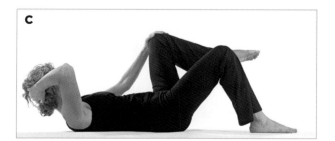

C. Exhale, and let your back come down to the mat. Then contract your abdominal muscles so that your lower back flattens on the floor, and lift up your head with your right hand.

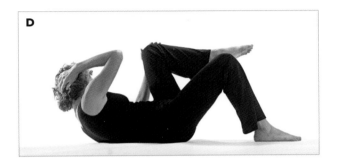

D. Tighten your abdominal muscles even more as you deeply round your back, and curl upward on the diagonal, pointing your right elbow toward your left knee. Contract your oblique muscles—the muscles on the side of your body, which you use to twist—to bring your elbow across your body.

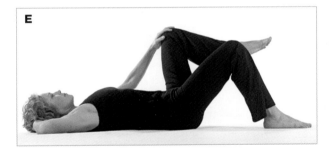

E. Slowly come back down as you lengthen your abdominals across the front of your body. Bring yourself back to neutral and relax your arms and back completely.

Repeat this movement 4–6 times on each side.

Diagonal Arch and Curl *(continued)*

NOTICE AND SENSE

The point of this movement is not to force your elbow to touch your knee. It is to coordinate the back and front of your body on a diagonal plane. As your front tightens and you curl up to reach your elbow across to your knee, your back muscles relax and lengthen on the diagonal to allow that to happen.

This movement is similar to the Back Lift movement (page 51), in which when you lift your opposing elbow and leg simultaneously. In this movement, you are lifting your opposing elbow and knee simultaneously.

Sense the diagonal lengthening from your hip across your chest to your armpit as you roll back down. Relax the front of your body gently and slowly.

If this bothers your neck, you are probably using your neck and shoulder muscles, not your abdominal muscles, to round up. When you have sensory motor amnesia, it's not uncommon to "recruit the neighbors" to get the job done: in other words, you're using muscles you don't need to use. Don't strain! Only go as far as is comfortable. *Go slowly*, and contract intentionally, in order to be sure you are engaging your abdominals and not your neck to do the movement.

After finishing this movement, lengthen your legs down, rest your arms alongside your body, and sense your back muscles. Sense whether they feel more relaxed on the floor. Breathe deeply into the center of your body. Sense the difference in your ability to breathe deeply.

6

The Flower

This movement helps to relax those muscles on the front of your body that, when habitually contracted, create stooped, hunched posture and shallow breathing. When you relax and lengthen these muscles, then you can stand taller and breathe more deeply. Do this movement as if you were yawning—opening first one side of the body, then the other.

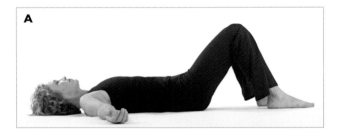

A. Lie on your back with your arms comfortably on the floor, resting slightly away from your body. This position keeps your shoulders more relaxed. Bring your knees up and plant your feet.

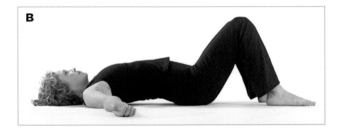

B. Inhale and gently arch your lower back as your tailbone tilts and rolls down in the direction of your feet. The lower back is gently arched; the front of your body is relaxed and open. Your neck is relaxed and long.

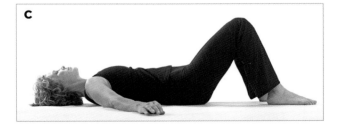

C. Exhale and slowly drop your back to the floor.

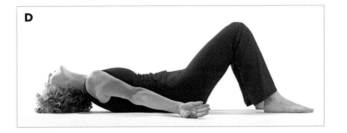

D. As your back flattens and your abdominals tighten, slowly roll your arms and hands inward toward your legs so that the backs of your hands are facing your thighs. Let your shoulders round up and in toward the midline of your body. Your neck gently arches and your chin tilts up toward the ceiling. You're tight on the entire front of your body. Even your inner thighs tighten.

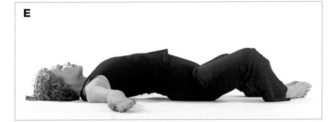

E. Inhale and reverse direction: the abdominals relax as you inhale and arch. Your shoulders roll out and open as your arms and hands roll out and away from your body. Allow your arms and hands to roll as far back and outward as they want. Let your shoulders relax and open as your arms roll away from the your body. At the same time, allow your legs to slowly open outward, and relax your inner thighs. The soles of your feet come together.

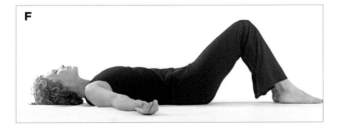

F. Exhale and slowly flatten your back, bringing your legs back together and bringing your arms back down to your sides.

Repeat this 4–6 times, slowly and easily. Make the movement nice and smooth.

NOTICE AND SENSE

Sense the difference in the front of your body between the times you inhale and move and the times when you exhale and move. When you inhale, your front is relaxed and long. Your legs are open. When you exhale, all the muscles in the front of your body contract and tighten. Think of this movement as if you were a flower: your back muscles arch as the petals open, and the front of your body rounds inward as they close.

Many of us, over time, can get stuck in a slumped, hunched posture. We may round inward when we're stressed, fearful or feeling anxious: this is the Red Light Reflex. This movement teaches you to create that reflex on purpose, then reverse it and relax all the muscles involved. This will help you become more skilled at self-correction if you notice that you're slumped. This will also help you control the muscles of breathing, which so often tighten when we're anxious or afraid. Maintaining the ability to breathe deeply is essential to overall good health.

This is an especially helpful movement if you work on a computer all day. You can even do it at your desk—rounding inward with your shoulders, arms, hands, and back, then opening outward, then returning to neutral. As with every movement in this book, try doing it as if you were yawning and just waking up in the morning.

7

Side Bend

This movement, which will help you stand taller and achieve better balance, addresses the waist muscles on the side of the body. When contracted, these muscles will pull your hip up and your ribs and shoulder down. Unconsciously holding yourself in this contracted position, with the waist muscles tight on one side, can adversely affect your balance in addition to causing a leg-length discrepancy, a rotation in the pelvis, and uneven shoulder height.

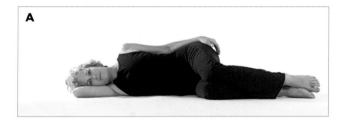

A. Lie on your right side with your legs at right angles to your waist, as if you were sitting in a straight-back chair.

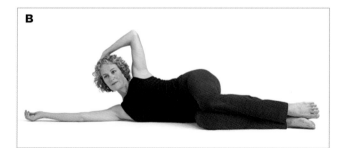

B. Bring your left arm over your head and grab the side of your head with your hand. Inhale and expand your ribs, then exhale and slowly lift your head. Feel your ribs contract as your waist tightens to bring your head up.

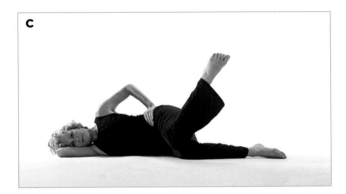

C. Place your hand on your hip bone so you can feel the movement of your hip. With your knees "glued" together, lift your top foot. Allow your hip to lift up and inward. Feel it with your hand. Your hip lifts and rolls upward and inward as your foot lifts. Slowly bring your leg and hip back down to a neutral position.

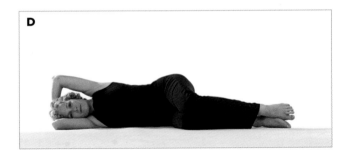

D. Now let's put both these movements together: first, bring your left arm over your head and grab the side of your head with your hand, as in step B. Then, focusing on the muscles of your waist, breathe in.

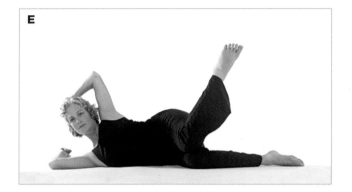

E. As you exhale, squeeze your ribs down in the direction of your waist as you lift your head up. At the same time, keeping your knees "glued" together, bring your top foot upward toward the ceiling. Sense the tightness in your waist! It's as if you were playing the accordion with your waist muscles. Your hip is tightening up toward your ribs while your ribs are tightening down toward your hip.

Come up only as far as is comfortable. Keep your head looking straight ahead so that you use the side of your body (the waist muscles) to do the work, not the front or back of your body.

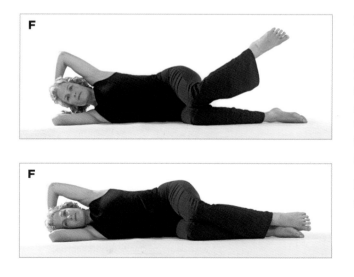

F. Slowly bring your foot and your head back down. Your hip comes back down and out to neutral as your foot lowers. Your ribs lift up and you lengthen through the waist as you bring your head down. Sense the relaxation and lengthening in the left side of your body as you breathe deeply.

Repeat this movement 3–5 times on each side.

NOTICE AND SENSE

Sense how your waist muscles tighten as you lift your head and foot to make an "accordion" out of the side of your body. Then sense how the entire side of your body lengthens as you bring your head and foot down. As you lengthen, gently lift your ribs up out of your waist as if you were reaching for something above your head. You are pandiculating the muscles on the side of your body by contracting into them, then releasing out of them.

Notice how, as you contract to bring your foot and head up, the opposite side of your body (the side against the floor) lengthens. Your ribs expand.

It is your waist muscles (the obliques), not your neck muscles, that contract to lift your head up off the floor. Tighten them deliberately so that your brain begins to notice how they move and can therefore deliberately lengthen and release them. If your neck bothers you when you do this movement, go more slowly, and try not to lift your head as high. It is always acceptable to do small "micromovements" until you regain awareness of the muscles.

If you have trouble and can't sense how to tighten and release your waist muscles, gently push a couple of fingers into the flesh between your ribs and pelvis, then slowly lift your foot and head at the same time. Do you feel a contraction under your fingers? You can also stand up and bend from side to side; that movement often brings more awareness of the waist muscles.

8

The Propeller

This movement is wonderful for lengthening the entire side of your body, from your shoulder all the way down to your hips. Relax in the center and allow your upper body to twist one way as your lower body twists the other way. This movement will also help you to breathe more deeply. As you reach the upper body alternately backward and forward, you relax and expand the rib cage for fuller, freer breathing. It's a completely natural movement. Do it slowly and luxuriously!

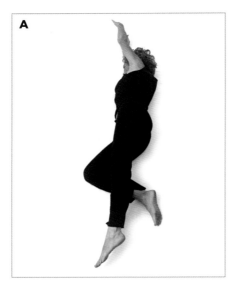

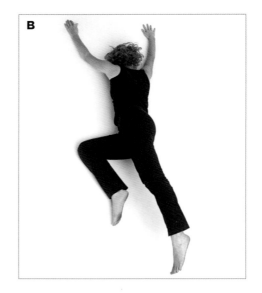

A. Lie on your right side and lay your head comfortably on your outstretched right arm. Bend your right knee a bit to stabilize yourself. Straighten your left leg down so that it is in line with your hip, and reach your left arm up over your head so that it is in line with your shoulder and hip. You are in one long line, like the blade of a propeller.

B. Inhale and reach forward with your left arm while you let your left leg move backward. Allow yourself to roll forward as you reach. If you let your pelvis roll slightly forward, this will allow you to reach your leg farther backward. Sense the nice long length along the left side of your body.

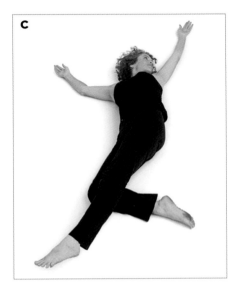

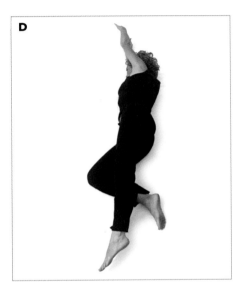

C. Reach as far backward with your left arm as is comfortable, as you allow your left leg to swing forward. Your upper body reaches backward as your leg swings forward. Follow your arm with your head and eyes. Let your hips roll back, and notice that this allows you to reach your leg forward. Allow your rib cage to open and lift. Inhale deeply. This is a smooth, rolling movement.

D. Bring your body back up to neutral with your arm, shoulder, hip, and leg in line with each other.

Reverse the movement by lying on your left side and reaching forward with your right arm and upper body while your right leg reaches backward. Then reach back with your arm and upper body, following your arm with your head, while your leg reaches forward. Repeat this several times.

The Propeller *(continued)*

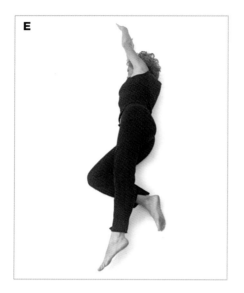

E. Bring your body back up to neutral with your arm, shoulder, hip, and leg in line with each other.

Reverse the movement by lying on your left side and reaching forward with your right arm and upper body while your right leg reaches backward. Then reach back with your arm and upper body, following your arm with your head, while your leg reaches forward. Repeat this several times.

NOTICE AND SENSE

Let your brain absorb the sensation of moving your upper body in one direction as your lower body moves in the other direction. This is a natural opposition—one that we use every day, especially when walking. Sense the length of your body from your armpit down along your rib cage and along the side of your waist, hip, and leg. Let your head move easily and smoothly.

9

The Washrag

In this movement you will experience the lengthening and releasing of your back, waist, and abdominal muscles as both your legs move one way and your head moves in the opposite direction. Your brain will absorb the feeling of a full-body lengthening and twisting; this will enable all the muscles at the center of your body to coordinate more smoothly.

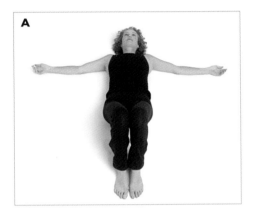

A. Bring your knees up and plant your feet near your buttocks. Place your arms straight out at your sides, palms up, as though you were forming a T. Let your elbows be loose; do not lock them.

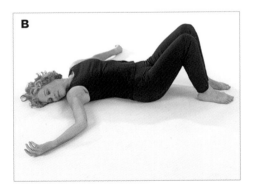

B. Begin by rotating your right arm, palm up, in the direction of your head while you rotate your left arm, palm down, in the direction of your feet. The sides of your palms will lift off the floor. Allow your head to gently roll toward the right.

The Washrag *(continued)*

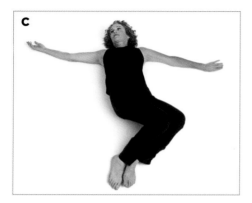

C. Now add the legs: allow both your legs to gently drop to the left as you continue to gently roll your head toward the right. Repeat this pattern several times until it feels comfortable: one arm rotates up as the other arm rotates down as your head turns toward the upturned arm.

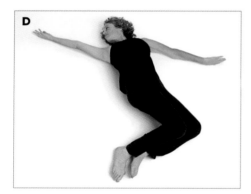

D. Continue to let your legs drop and lengthen as far as is comfortable. Don't push beyond your comfort range! This isn't a stretch—it's a conscious, controlled pandiculation—contracting, then lengthening . . . like a nice yawn!

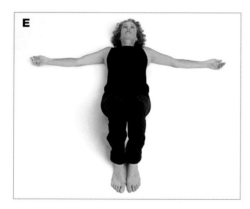

E. Inhale and slowly bring your legs back up to neutral. Notice the muscles in the center of your body that work to help you bring your legs up: your back drops back to the mat, your abdominals tighten, and your hip rotates back to neutral.

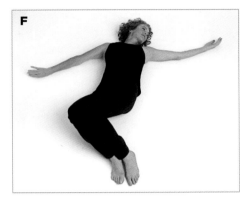

F. Now reverse direction: rotate your left arm, palm up, in the direction of your head while you rotate your right arm, palm down, in the direction of your feet. Allow your head to gently roll toward the left. Then allow both your legs to gently drop to the right as you continue to smoothly roll your head toward the left.

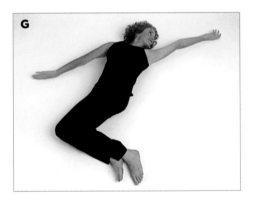

G. Continue this movement, your arms rotating gently in opposite directions as your legs flop over in opposition to your head. You're wringing yourself out, as you would wring out a washrag!

The Washrag *(continued)*

As you rotate your arm with your hand and palm up, your shoulder presses down into the floor or mat. As you rotate your arm with your hand and palm down, your shoulder rolls up off the floor or mat. Notice the gentle twisting of your shoulders in opposite directions. Allow your shoulders to move along with the movement. Let your elbows be loose and floppy rather than rigid and straight. The most natural way to turn your head is toward the upturned arm. You're twisting and lengthening at the same time. As your legs lengthen to one side, notice how the waist muscles on the other side of your body shorten. This is normal and natural.

As you lengthen and release your legs down to the floor or mat, you're creating a wonderful twist—what Hanna called a spiral twist; it is a natural, familiar movement for all of us. It's what happens when we walk: our shoulders and hips move in opposition to each other in order to counterbalance the weight of our swinging limbs.

Enjoy this somewhat sensuous movement, which lengthens your entire spine and center, all the way up through your shoulders and into your neck. Remember to relax your back, waist, buttocks, and abdominal muscles in order to twist more easily. Only go as far as is comfortable!

10

Hip Hikes

Now that you've learned to relax and release the muscles at the center of your body—the back, the abdominals, and the waist—you're ready to move your hips. The deep muscles of your back, once they're lengthened and under the brain's control, help to coordinate movement of the hips and pelvis. If your back and waist muscles remain tight and forget how to move, your pelvis becomes locked and immobile.

Learning to move your hips up and down, which I like to call hiking the hips, is something too many of us unlearn as we get older. I've noticed that those who continue to enjoy dancing are the ones who never forget that hips are for moving!

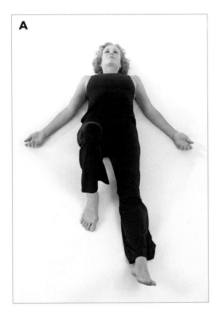

A

A. Begin on your back with your right knee up and your right foot planted near your buttocks. Straighten your left leg down on the floor. Your hips should be relaxed and "square" on the floor. Place your arms at your sides, slightly away from your body.

Hip Hikes *(continued)*

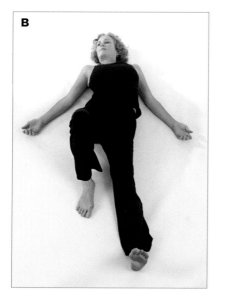

B. Gently tighten—or "hike"—your right hip upward in the direction of your armpit. Feel your waist muscles tighten on one side as you lengthen the muscles on the other side. As you hike, the sacrum and pelvis turn like a steering wheel. This is similar to the movement you did in the Side Bend (page 62).

Make sure your back is relaxed on the floor and that it doesn't arch in order to "help out." Your hip is sliding along the floor or mat as it hikes.

Relax your hip back down to neutral. Then change sides: bring your left knee up, plant your left foot, and straighten your right leg down. Slowly hike your left hip, and then relax it back to neutral. Repeat this movement several times on each side.

NOTICE AND SENSE

This movement, which addresses what Hanna called the vertical dimension of walking, should be done smoothly and gently. Don't push or force anything. Notice that, when one hip hikes up, the waist muscles on that side get tighter—and the waist muscles on the other side get longer. Pay as much attention to the side that lengthens as to the side that shortens, and notice that your brain naturally coordinates the movement as a whole. If you've ever danced, this will be a familiar and fun movement. Remembering to allow the hips to swing a little when you walk will make walking much easier.

11

Human X

This movement helps you to sense how a relaxed center of the body allows for more movement in your arms and legs. If you're tight in the center—in the waist, abdominals, and back—your ability to reach with and lengthen your arms and legs is restricted. Remember to relax and release the center of your body before beginning this movement.

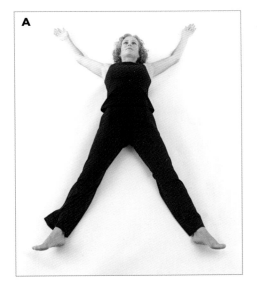

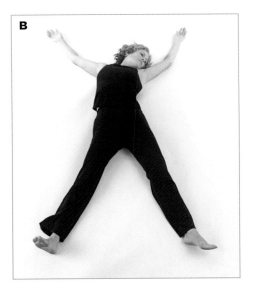

A. Lie on your back and bring your arms up above your head, slightly wider than shoulder width apart. Open your legs slightly wider than hip width apart, so that your body now looks like an X. If your shoulders and chest are tight and it's difficult to put your arms on the floor above your head, you can prop your arms up on pillows above your head.

B. Slowly reach downward with your right leg. Then bring it back to neutral and relax. Do this lazily, like a marionette being pulled one string at a time.

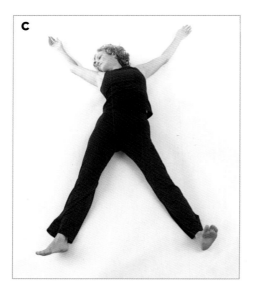

C. Now reach downward with your left leg. Then bring it back to neutral and relax. Notice the lengthening of your left side and the shortening of your right side.

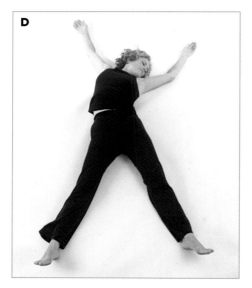

D. Now reach up with your right arm—slowly and lazily, just as you did with your legs. Bring your arm back to neutral and relax. Again, notice how reaching and lengthening on one side shortens the other side.

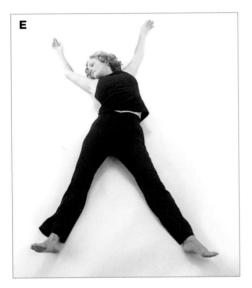

E. Now reach up with your left arm, then bring it back and relax. Enjoy that nice relaxation in the center of your body. Notice once more that your right side shortened as your left side lengthened.

Repeat this pattern 4–5 times—right leg, left leg, right arm, left arm.

NOTICE AND SENSE

This movement addresses all the muscles of the trunk—the obliques, the extensors, and the flexors. It encourages you to relax and then release them, instead of tightening them as we so often do in our daily lives. Notice that the more you relax the center of your body, the farther you can extend each leg and each arm. Practicing the X pattern also brings an awareness of the waist muscles by getting your hips moving up and down, alternately lengthening and shortening the muscles as you go. This is extremely important for increasing flexibility in the pelvis, which in turn promotes smoother, easier walking. This movement helps even out leg length, too. Do this movement as if you were just waking up in the morning and "yawning out" your limbs. It feels great!

12

Inversion and Eversion of the Feet

This movement helps you to sense and improve the coordination among your feet, knees, hips, and back. The more relaxed you are in the center of your body, the easier it is to move these parts together.

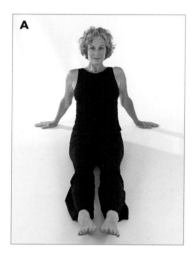

A. Sit up on the floor with your legs straight out in front of you. Lean back slightly and support yourself with your arms behind you.

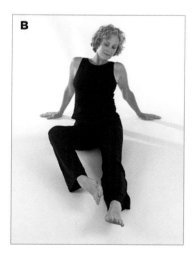

B. Turn your right foot inward and gently up toward your face, as though you're checking to see if there's something on the bottom of your right foot. Let your right knee bend and drop outward as your foot turns inward and your ankle bends. You are now inverting your foot. In inversion, the foot turns inward, the knee drops outward, and the hip opens up and allows the knee to descend outward. Notice how the left side of your back arches slightly when you invert your foot.

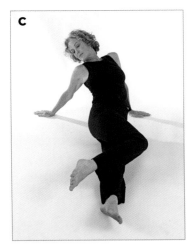

C. Now "wing" your foot outward, and lift your right hip slightly off the floor as you turn your torso to the left. Allow your right knee to drop and cross over your left knee. Turn your head gently to the right to check whether you can see whatever's on the bottom of your foot from this angle. You are now everting your foot. In eversion, the foot turns outward and the knee drops inward and over the opposite knee—almost as if you're kicking something away from you. Notice how the right side of your back arches in order to help you with the movement.

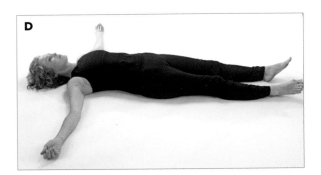

D. Now let's try it another way. Lie on your back with your legs straight down on the floor. Position your arms straight out from your shoulders, as though you were forming a T.

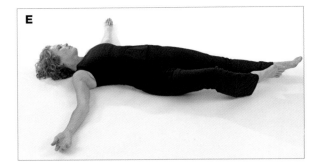

E. Invert your right foot and lift it off the floor slightly. Slowly draw it up alongside your left leg. Gently press into the floor or mat with your left shoulder. Let your knee drop out as your hip begins to open. Let the left side of your back begin to arch.

Inversion and Eversion of the Feet *(continued)*

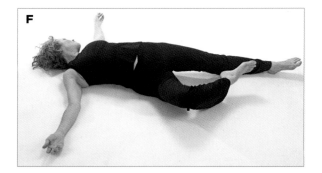

F. Continue to draw your foot upward toward your left knee. Let your right knee continue to drop, your right hip continue to open, and the left side of your back arch further. Your entire body is gently twisting. Sense the weight in your right hip. Allow your head to turn in the direction as your foot is pointing.

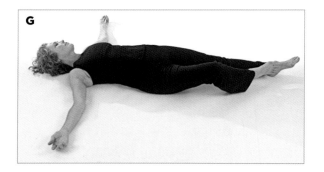

G. Slowly bring your foot back down, sliding it along the inside of your left leg. Your back will lengthen and relax to the floor, your hip will come back to neutral, your knee will turn inward, and your leg will straighten. Make this movement as smooth as possible.

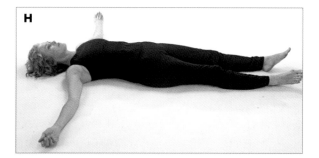

H. Relax back to neutral.

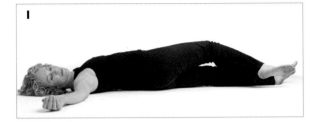

I. Evert your right foot and lift it slightly off the floor. Your knee will drop inward toward your left leg, your foot will point outward away from your body, and your right hip will lift off the floor.

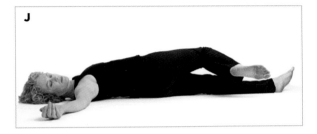

J. Draw your right foot up farther, as if you want to see the bottom of your foot. Allow your right knee to drop farther over your left leg. Your right hip will lift and turn, and the right side of your back will arch and lengthen, to aid the movement. Allow your head to turn in the same direction as your foot.

K. Slowly bring your foot back down. Your back will lengthen, your hip will rotate back to neutral, your right knee will turn back to the center, and your leg will straighten out.

Inversion and Eversion of the Feet *(continued)*

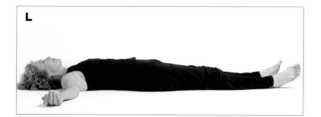

L. Bring your leg and foot back down to the floor and completely relax.

Repeat this sequence 3–4 times on each side. Turn your foot inward (invert it), draw it up toward the inside of the opposite knee, and drop your knee as your hip opens. Let the opposite side of your back arch, and let your head look in the same direction as your foot is pointing. Bring your leg down slowly to neutral. Then turn your foot out (evert it), drop your knee to the inside, lift your hip, and arch your back on the same side, as your head turns in the same direction as your foot. Bring your leg down to neutral and relax.

NOTICE AND SENSE

Notice the connection between your foot, knee, hip, and back: the movement of your foot moves your knee, which moves your hip, which in turn moves your back. They can all move beautifully together when you let them. When done in one smooth motion, this movement can help relieve soreness in your feet, knees, and hips.

In order to do this movement, it's essential that you release your back and allow it to arch and twist in order to facilitate opening and closing your hip. Remember that you're training your brain to regain sensory awareness and control of these very natural movements of the body. You're becoming more body-intelligent in order to achieve better physical coordination.

13

Skiing

This movement takes the inversion-eversion concept just a bit further. Notice whether this movement's full-body turning and twisting motion gives you more awareness of your feet, legs, hips, and back.

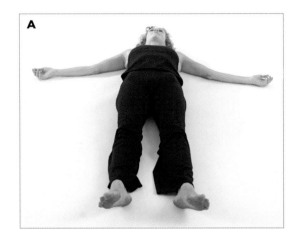

A. Lie on your back with your legs straight and your arms positioned at right angles to your sides. Keep your knees and elbows loose and unlocked.

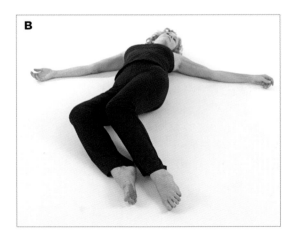

B. Slowly invert (turn in) your right foot and evert (turn out) your left foot. Allow your back and hips to follow your knees as they drop to the right.

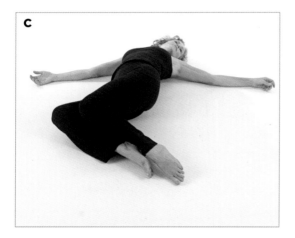

C. Slowly bring your feet up farther toward your head, and allow your knees to drop farther to the right. Your back will arch gently toward the same side as the turned-out foot. Let this happen. Feel the twisting and turning of your feet, knees, hips, and torso. Enjoy it—it's as if you were skiing!

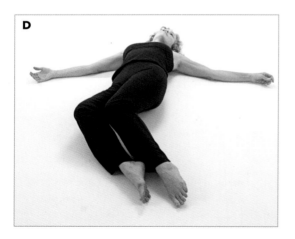

D. Slowly bring your knees back to the center, ease your back down to the floor, and straighten your legs.

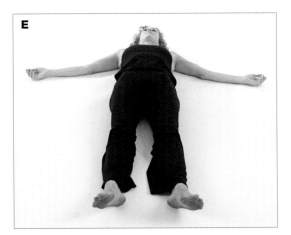

E. Relax completely, with your legs straight and your back in a neutral position on the floor.

Repeat the movement 5–6 times on each side—alternating from your right side to your left side—and imagine that you're skiing slowly down a mountain!

NOTICE AND SENSE

Sense how much more flexibility you have in your feet, knees, hips, and legs after doing this movement. The flexibility comes not only from the relaxation in the center of your body, but also from your legs and feet, which should be freer, more relaxed, and more under the brain's control after you learn the inversion-eversion technique. Experiencing the way in which the movement of your feet affects your knees, hips, and back can make many daily activities seem effortless.

14

Steeple Twist

This fun movement relaxes the muscles of the trunk and hips. It will further enhance your ability to rotate the center of your body as you release the muscles involved in the Trauma Reflex. It will also help keep your spine flexible. The gentle twisting of the spine is an essential human movement, integral to many daily activities, including walking and running.

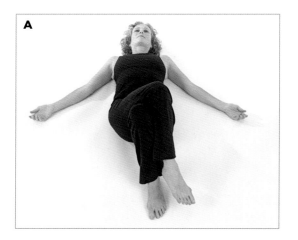

A. Lie on your back with your knees up and your feet planted near your buttocks. Then cross your right leg over your left leg. Position your arms at a 45-degree angle away from your body.

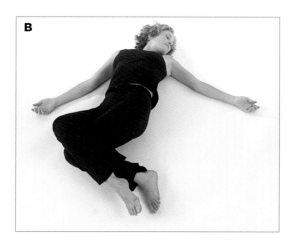

B. Inhale, then, as you exhale, allow the weight of your top leg to bring both legs down to the right. Make sure to relax your chest muscles, abdominal muscles, and the waist muscles on your left side. Go only as far as is comfortable without forcing. Let your head roll to the left as your legs go to the right.

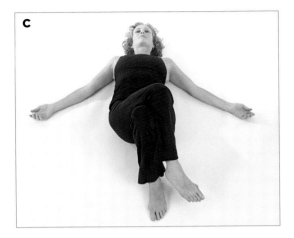

C. Inhale, and, using all the muscles of your trunk as you exhale, bring your knees back up to neutral.

Repeat steps A–C 6–8 times on the right side, sensing the lengthening of the left side of your body from your armpit down across your chest and into your hip and groin. This pandiculates the muscles of your trunk as you contract them to bring your legs up and release them as you bring your legs down.

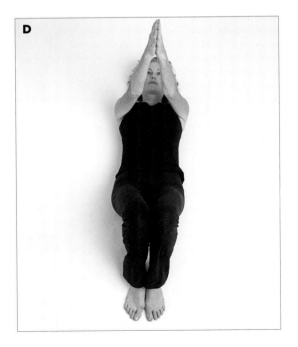

D. Uncross your knees and, keeping your knees vertical, plant your feet near your buttocks. Put both palms together, as though you were forming a steeple. Keep your arms straight and point them up to the ceiling. Imagine that you have Krazy Glue® on your palms. Keep your elbows straight.

Steeple Twist *(continued)*

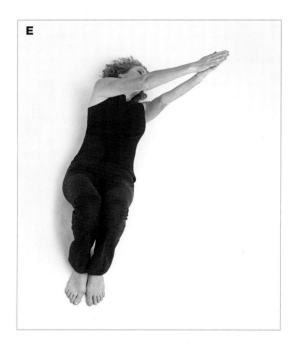

E. Inhale and tilt the "steeple" over to the left. Make sure to let your head and eyes turn and follow your hands. As your arms tilt, your right shoulder will lift and you'll put more weight into your left shoulder. Go only as far as is comfortable, keeping your elbows straight and your hands together. Your knees should stay vertical while your upper trunk turns. Repeat this three times slowly.

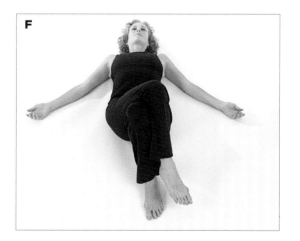

F. Bring your arms and hands down to a neutral position on the floor and relax. Cross your right leg over your left leg once again.

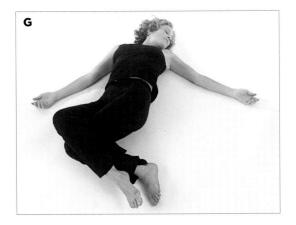

G

G. Inhale, and, as you exhale, allow your legs to drop over to the right, going only as far as is comfortable. Notice whether you have increased your range of motion after having focused on twisting your upper body.

Repeat steps A–G on the left side. Notice the difference between your ability to move your legs and hips on the left side and your ability to move them on the right side.

NOTICE AND SENSE

When we walk, our shoulders and hips should move gently in opposition. This happens in the steeple twist as the hips go one way and the upper body goes the other way.

As you twist, notice the lengthening across your chest and ribs and up into your neck. You'll feel release in your buttocks and in the sides of your legs as well. Each time you do this movement, see if you can notice something new. Challenge yourself to go slowly and make the movement as smooth as possible. As you tilt your "steeple arms," sense the lengthening deep into your back as you tilt your arms over to the side. Notice the difference between your ability to tilt over to one side as compared to the other.

If your legs went farther down to the side after you isolated your upper body with the steepled-arm movement, it was because you were *differentiating* your upper body from your lower body. You were also doing a movement your brain isn't used to. This brings it greater stimulation and feedback, which, in turn, increases your range of motion without force.

15

Seated Twist

This exercise is wonderful for freeing the muscles in your neck and shoulders. It was developed by the late somatic educator Moshe Feldenkrais. As you focus on each small muscle group that takes part in the larger movement, your range of motion increases and those individual muscles become freer.

This movement is also a perfect example of the fact that changing your brain's neurological patterns increases your awareness of and control over your physical and muscular patterns—all without forcing or stretching.

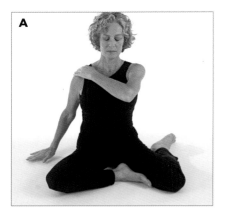

A. Sit on the floor with your knees bent, your right leg turned out and your right foot inverted, and your left leg turned in and your left foot everted. Put the sole of your right foot on your left thigh. Support yourself with your right hand at your side. If you can keep your torso vertical, with your weight on both buttocks, that's best. However, if you need to lean on your supporting hand and your left buttock comes off the floor, that's okay, too. Place your left hand on your right shoulder. Lift your left elbow slightly. This helps to open your shoulder. You're facing what we're going to call the front. Close your eyes.

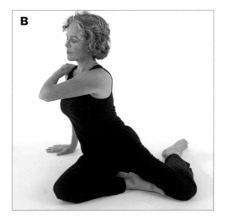

B. Slowly twist around in the direction of your right shoulder, as far as is comfortable.

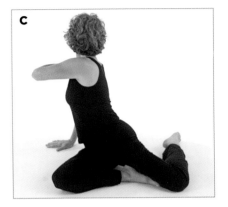

C. Continue to twist around so that you're facing the opposite direction—180 degrees from the point at which you started, or as far as is comfortable. We'll call this the back. Then slowly reverse direction and twist around so that you're facing front again. Do this three times slowly. On the third time, stop when you're facing the back, or at your comfortable limit, and open your eyes. Make a mental note of something in the room that lets you know where your present limit is.

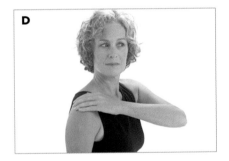

D. Keeping your torso where it is, and without moving your head, slowly look to the left, then to the right. Moving only your eyes, repeat this movement four times. Notice everything in your line of your vision. Then slowly bring your entire body back to the front.

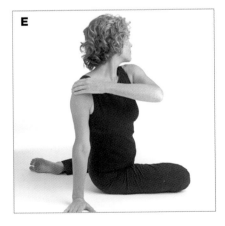

E. Inhale and twist around to your limit and stop. Keep your body where it is and, moving just your head and eyes, look to the left.

Seated Twist *(continued)*

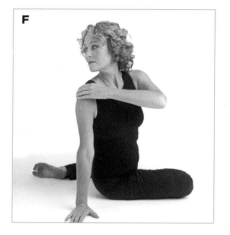

F. Slowly turn your head and eyes in the opposite direction, and look to the right. Repeat that neck movement four times slowly. Notice the sensations in your neck and eyes. The neck muscles may quiver as you concentrate on slowly moving the eyes together with the neck. That's okay. Notice everything in your line of vision as you turn your head. Then slowly bring your entire body back to the front.

Close your eyes, inhale, and twist around to the back three times. On the third time, open your eyes and see how much farther you can twist.

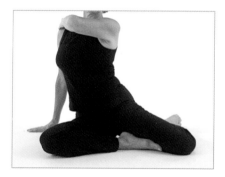

Variation 1

Sit in the same position as in step A. Close your eyes. Bring your awareness to your left hip. Lift your hip up and down a couple of times. Then, as you twist around toward the right, intentionally lift your left hip again. Make it part of the entire turning movement. Come back to the front.

Repeat this movement three times: inhale, lift your hip, twist around to your limit, open your left ribs and left shoulder blade, and slowly turn your head to the right and left. On the last turn, stop and open your eyes. Notice how you've increased your range of motion by lifting your hip.

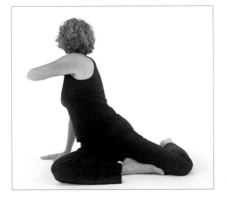

Variation 2

Sit in the same position as in step A. Keeping your eyes open, inhale and twist all the way around and stop. Keep your body turned to the back as you turn your head to your left shoulder. Then turn your body to the front as you bring your head to your right shoulder.

Repeat this variation 3–5 times, slowly and smoothly. This is a brainteaser, but you're beginning to create more complex movement challenges for your brain.

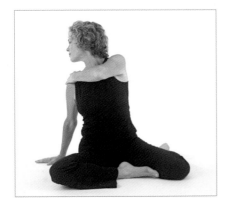

Finally, close your eyes, and twist around to the back three times. On the third time, open your eyes, and see how far you've come!

Repeat the entire series of movements, including the variations, on the other side. Feel free to choose different variations for each side just to give your brain more stimulation and feedback.

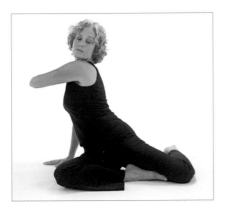

Seated Twist *(continued)*

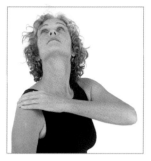 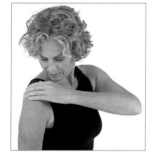

Variation 3

Sit in the same position as in step A. Keeping your eyes open, inhale and twist around to your limit. Moving just your head, slowly look up to the ceiling. Then slowly look down. Move your eyes along with your head. Repeat the slow nodding four times. Then slowly come back around to the front.

Repeat the entire movement with your eyes closed—inhale, twist around, stop at your limit—then open your eyes and notice how far you've come.

NOTICE AND SENSE

With each variation, how much more range of motion did you achieve?

Each time you consciously bring in a new variation or area of awareness to this movement, you give the brain more information about how to coordinate all the muscles involved. You are differentiating the movements: the eyes from the head; the neck from the shoulders and hips. When you put it all together, the movement is not only smoother, but you are able to go much farther than the first time you tried it!

Sense each element involved in this pattern: the lifting of the hip; the opening of the rib cage; the turning of the shoulder, neck, and head; and then finally the movement of the eyes. We're so accustomed to moving our bodies as one solid unit that we forget that full-body movement is made up of many smaller parts.

16

Walking Lessons

Now we can put to good use much of the coordination we achieved when we worked on twisting, hip hikes, and releasing and lengthening the back. These movements simulate the normal mechanics of walking while "out of gravity," so that when you're back up "in gravity"—standing—you can create a new, more fluid pattern of walking.

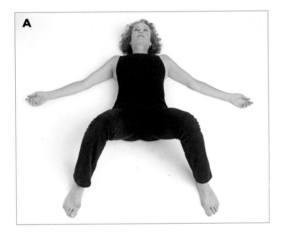

A. Lie on your back with your knees up and feet planted wide apart. Relax your arms at a 45-degree angle away from your body.

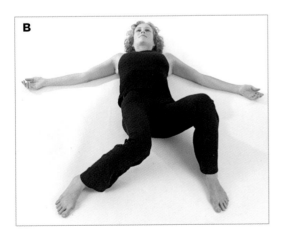

B. Slowly reach your right knee inward toward your left heel. Let your back and waist muscles on the right side relax as your pelvis rolls slightly. As your knee drops inward, you will roll on the inside of your foot. Keep your shoulders on the floor or mat.

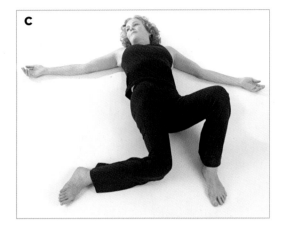

C. Reach your knee and leg inward as far as is comfortable. Your knee moves inward, but also downward. This lengthens the waist, back, and abdominal muscles. Let your pelvis roll to allow the movement to occur. Repeat this slowly 5–8 times.

No stretching allowed! Only go as far as is comfortable, then bring your knee back up to neutral.

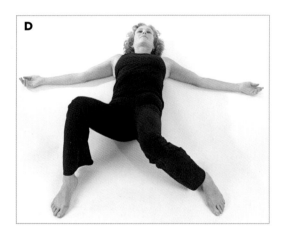

D. Repeat the same movement 5–8 times on the left. Relax your back and gently reach your left knee and leg inward toward your right heel.

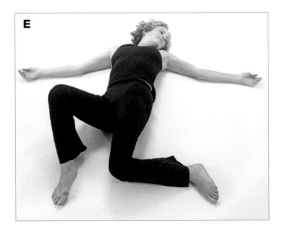

E. Allow your back to lengthen and your left hip to roll forward and upward. This allows your leg and knee to reach downward toward your right heel. Make sure to enjoy the rolling movement of your pelvis!

Bring your knee back up to neutral. Now alternate between right and left: your right knee goes down, and back up, then your left knee goes down and back up. Let your back relax as you roll your pelvis. Let your foot roll to the inside as your knee comes down and inward. If it feels relaxed and smooth, you can speed it up a little, just for fun! Enjoy flopping your legs back and forth, just as you might have done when you were a child.

NOTICE AND SENSE

Notice that your hip joint and pelvis can't roll if your back or abdominal muscles are tight. That's because this movement comes from your back rather than your legs. If the center of your body is tight, your pelvis won't relax and rock, and you won't be able to drop your knee and leg down in the direction of the opposite heel.

Sense your pelvis rolling like a barrel as one leg comes down, then up, and the other leg comes down, then up. You should feel a smooth rolling on your sacrum as you do this movement. Notice that when you reach one leg down, the opposite side of your waist contracts. This is what happens when we walk. Don't be afraid to rock and roll!

17

Walking Lessons Part 2

Now we'll expand on the walking-lesson movement you just learned. Recall the sensation of allowing your back to lengthen and your pelvis to roll as you dropped your knee and leg inward. Keep that awareness as you take your knee and leg forward in this next movement.

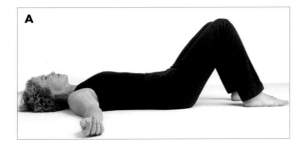

A. Lie on your back with both knees up and your feet planted near your buttocks.

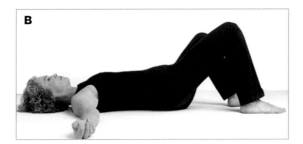

B. Press down with your right foot, and push your right knee and thigh straight forward while lifting your hip to allow the movement to happen. Your back will arch slightly and the entire right side of your body will lengthen. This is what you did when you dropped your knee inward, only this time your knee is going forward.

Bring your knee and leg back to neutral. Your hip joint will return to the floor.

Repeat this movement 4–6 times.

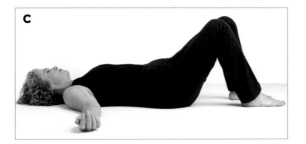

C. Now do the same movement with the other leg: Press down into the floor with your left foot as you push your left knee and thigh forward and allow your hip and pelvis to lift and roll. The entire right side of your body—the waist, ribs, back, and abdominals—lengthens and releases. Remember to keep your left foot planted.

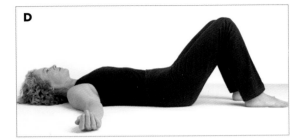

D. Bring your knee, thigh, and hip back to neutral.

Repeat this movement 4–6 times on this side.

Now alternate: first push your right knee and thigh forward, then your left knee and thigh. Remember to let your pelvis roll!

NOTICE AND SENSE

This movement addresses the horizontal (backward-and-forward) aspect of walking, whereas the hip hikes address the vertical (up-and-down) aspect of walking. As it does in the "knee dropping inward" movement you did previously, your pelvis rolls like a barrel in order to let your knee and thigh reach forward. Think of the coordination inherent in running: as your leg reaches forward to take a stride, your hip slightly twists forward and your back releases to aid in the movement. Also, when one knee pushes forward and the same side of your body lengthens, your hip contracts on the other side and shortens naturally. Again, this is what should happen with easy, relaxed walking.

If you're having difficulty sensing the rolling and twisting of your pelvis, lie on the floor and place your hands on your pelvic bones. Lift one hip up toward the ceiling as you shift your weight to the other hip, then bring the raised hip back down to the floor. Now lift the other hip and bring it down slowly. Once you get the feeling of rocking that comes from lifting one hip up, then the other, speed up the movement slightly. You're rolling like a barrel on your sacrum and hips.

18

Seated Mirror Study

Do you have chronic lower back pain, or neck and shoulder pain? Do you sit all day at your job? It could be that the way in which you "sit up straight" contributes to your discomfort more than you realize. This movement will help you sit in a more balanced way. It will also you become more self-correcting should you begin to feel discomfort while sitting.

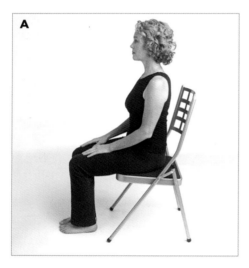

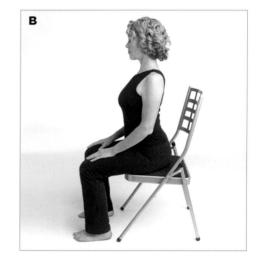

A. Sit on a firm, nonupholstered chair next to a full-length mirror. Don't face the mirror directly—sit so that you can see yourself in profile in the mirror. Sit with your back in a relaxed, neutral position, as shown in the photo. Your spine should be supported and balanced over your pelvis, and your back should be relaxed.

B. Now arch your back and push your chest forward slightly. This is one of the two versions of "straight" that I see most often—your back is arched and your weight is pitched forward. This is a typical Green Light Reflex pose— ready to move on and get things done. It pulls the spine into a bow rather than allowing it to be vertical and relaxed. The back muscles contract from the tailbone all the way up to the base of the neck. It's a very common posture for those who work with computers all day long.

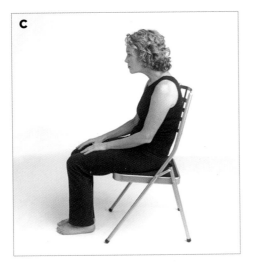

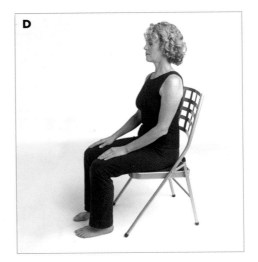

C. Now slump back into the chair so that your back touches the backrest. Slightly hunch your shoulders. This is the other version of "straight" I often see—the exact opposite of the green light posture. Your belly is tight, your weight rests on the back of your pelvis, and your neck juts forward. This can create a tight, painful neck and a sore upper back.

Whichever way you sit—arched forward or rounded down—either extreme is uncomfortable. In time, your body comes to accept these extremes as the norm. After all, your muscles are simply doing what you tell them to do.

D. Now close your eyes and sit up to what feels "straight" for you. Then open your eyes and look in the mirror. Are you arched? Rounded? What's your "norm?" Notice how you feel, but don't try to change it. Now close your eyes again.

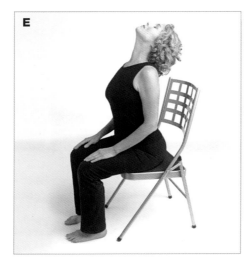

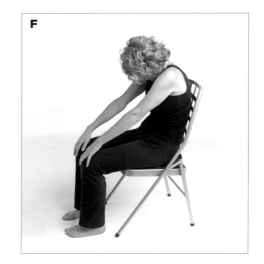

E. Keeping your eyes closed, inhale and slowly arch your back gently as you look up to the ceiling. Let your pelvis tilt forward as your back arches. Let the front of your body be relaxed, long, and open.

F. Exhale and slowly round your lower back and let your pelvis curl under slightly. Let your head drop down. Curl inward through the center of your body.

Repeat this arching and rounding pattern 2–3 times. Make the movement slow and smooth. Let your pelvis rock back and forth. Let your head go back as you arch your back. Let your head drop down as you round forward.

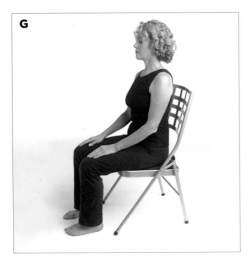

G. Now slowly come up to what your brain tells you is straight.

Keeping your eyes closed, sense your back and spine. Are they on top of your sit bones? Are they in front? In back? Do some self-adjustment. Relax your buttocks. Rock slowly from side to side on your sit bones. Touch your hip flexors at the groin line. Are they relaxed? When you feel relaxed and balanced, open your eyes. See if your internal sensations agree with what you see in the mirror. If you're still arched or rounded, close your eyes and do it again. The goal is to get your internal sense of "straight" to agree with your visual sense.

NOTICE AND SENSE

This exercise can permanently change the way in which you sit. With practice, you'll be able to sit effortlessly, without fatigue. You are retraining your internal awareness to agree with what you see in the mirror. At first you might feel slumped or out of balance. Don't worry. Your brain has created a habit that needs to be changed slowly but surely. Eventually, slumping or overarching will feel odd and uncomfortable instead of normal.

19

Side Bend Mirror Study

This movement helps you achieve a more accurate sense of what it means to be balanced and symmetrical on both sides of your body.

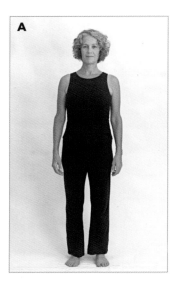

A. Stand in front of a full-length mirror and notice how you look. Are your shoulders balanced? Does one shoulder look lower than the other? What about your arms? Does one of them look longer than the other? Are you standing with equal weight on both feet? Now close your eyes, stand in a position that you feel is normal, and notice how you feel.

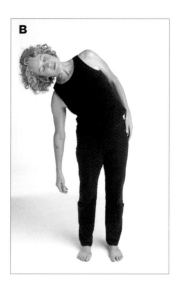

B. With your eyes closed, inhale and bend slowly over to your right side. Make sure you're going to the side and not twisting to the back or front. Inhale deeply and sense your ribs expanding on the left side as your waist muscles lengthen to allow you to bend. Notice your waist muscles tightening on the right side.

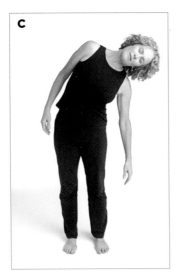

C. Keeping your eyes closed, exhale, come slowly up to neutral, and bend over to the left side. As you bend, inhale deeply and feel your ribs expand on the right side. Your waist lengthens on the right side as your ribs tighten and squeeze down on the left side. Repeat one more time, bending to the left, then slowly over to the right.

Exhale, come back up to neutral, and sense how your weight is distributed. Your eyes are still closed. Are you balanced? Sense both sides of your ribs and waist. Is one side more relaxed than the other? Are you standing with your weight equally on both feet? Do your shoulders feel level? Sense a lengthening on both sides of your body. When you think you're symmetrical and balanced, open your eyes. If you see that one shoulder is pulled down or that you're tilted to one side, close your eyes and repeat steps A–C until you can come up to a balanced neutral position.

NOTICE AND SENSE

As you bend, let go of your shoulders. Sense the muscles on the side of your body tightening and lengthening as you bend from side to side. These are the muscles that allow your torso to lean, not the muscles in your shoulders. For more sensory awareness, you can place a hand on the side of your ribs as you inhale and tilt to one side. Feel your ribs expand under your hand as that side lengthens.

As with all the somatic movements you're doing, you are retraining your brain to help you achieve better muscle control and proprioception. By having an accurate internal awareness of your body, and by retraining your muscles to agree with what you see in the mirror, you will be better able to self-adjust and self-monitor without the mirror.

20

Posture Pillow

Remember the old-fashioned exercise in which young girls put books on their heads in order to achieve good posture? Well, in many places outside the U.S., people routinely carry heavy loads on their heads. I saw female construction workers in India carrying bricks on their heads, and women with piles of dish towels on their heads on their way to market in Africa. Although there can be risks involved in carrying heavy loads on one's head, this activity results in excellent posture and body mechanics. I saw very few people with rounded shoulders and hunched backs in either India or Africa.

However, in the beginning, be careful not to put anything heavier than a pillow on your own head for this movement. Carrying heavy loads before you've mastered the technique could cause your neck muscles to contract and possibly result in a painful injury.

One thing this movement teaches you is that it's impossible to carry a heavy load on your head (heavy or light) if your hips are tight and don't sway. Just as an earthquake-proof building gently sways during a tremor, our bodies are supposed to move freely, twisting slightly as we walk or run. This promotes coordinated, efficient movement and allows the joints to act as effective shock absorbers. Moving with a rigid torso, which some people advocate to protect a painful back, can actually contribute to back pain!

To prepare for the movement on page 107, lie down on the floor and relax. Breathe deeply and sense the center of your body. Do this for about a minute. Then stand up and notice what it feels like to stand. Where is the weight distributed when you stand? How do your ribs feel? Are they open and relaxed, or are they tight? Do your shoulders feel even?

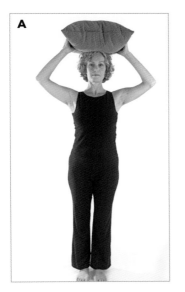

A. Remain standing and put a pillow on top of your head. Hold it gently on both sides with your elbows out and up. Notice your ribs. Breathe deeply and lift your ribs gently. Is it easier to lift your chest when you have something on your head? Sense how your abdominal muscle lengthens and supports your center.

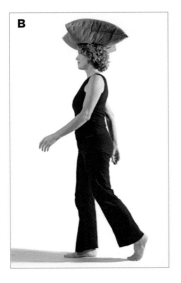

B. Walk slowly, letting your hips sway and rotate gently. How much taller do you feel? Walk for several minutes, then remove the pillow, lie down, and sense the center of your body. Breathe deeply. Are there differences between the way you feel now and the way you felt before you put the pillow on your head? Take that awareness into your day and see how it affects your movement.

21

The Shrug

Over the past few years, there have been many occasions when friends or clients will call and say, "I'm in terrible pain, but I can't get to you" (or "I'm on vacation," or "I'm in the office," or "I'm on the train . . ."). They ask, "Is there something I can do at home to relieve my pain?"

The answer to that question is always an emphatic yes! If you've read this far, you already know that simply by practicing the movements in this book every day—thus becoming more aware of your own internal sensations and the way in which you move—you will be less likely to experience chronic muscle pain.

But how do you remember the techniques you've learned in the moment when you are in pain?

Let's use a complaint common to many of my clients: a painful, tight, "I must have slept wrong" shoulder. Often, this condition involves the muscles along the top of the shoulder and down the bony part of the shoulder blade in back. The chest muscle—which attaches into the top of the upper arm at the front of the shoulder—is often a culprit, too.

For simplicity's sake, think of this movement as a gesture toward the four cardinal points of a compass: north, south, east, and west. This image will also help take your mind off your pain.

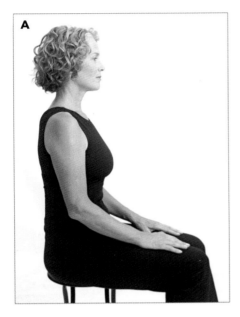

A. Sit on a firm, nonupholstered chair next to a full-length mirror. Don't face the mirror directly—sit so that you can see yourself in profile in the mirror. Sit with your back in a relaxed, neutral position, as shown in the photo. Your spine should be supported and balanced over your pelvis, and your back should be relaxed.

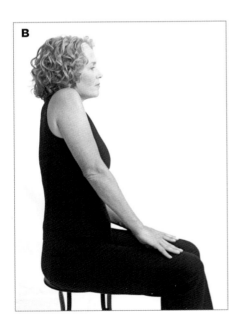

B. Draw your shoulder up toward your ear, then slowly bring it back to neutral. When you draw your shoulder up, you are tightening the muscle tighter than it already is, creating a pandicular response. Repeat this four times slowly.

Notice that when you tighten your shoulder up toward your ear, you open your torso through the ribs. Make sure your movements are smooth, not bumpy or jerky.

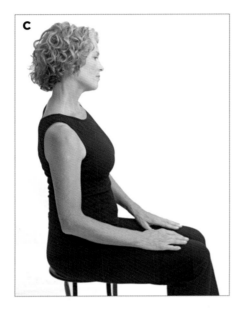

C. Draw your shoulder down past neutral, in the direction of your waist, and then slowly bring it back up to neutral. Repeat four times.

Notice that when you depress your shoulder, your ribs on that side also squeeze down. When you slowly bring your shoulder back to neutral, your ribs release and relax. The movement of the shoulder involves the center of the body!

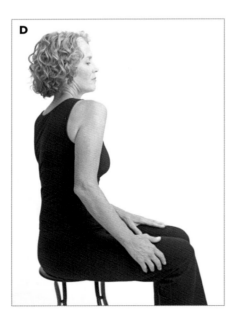

D. Slowly tighten your shoulder forward and inward, then slowly bring it back to neutral. Repeat four times.

Notice your chest muscle tightening as it draws your shoulder forward. Notice how your shoulder opens in back. Your chest muscle releases and relaxes when you bring your shoulder back to neutral.

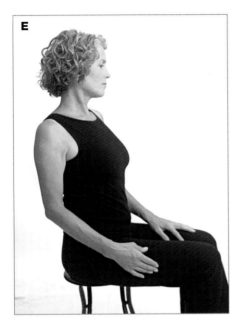

E. Slowly tighten your shoulder backward and gently squeeze the muscles in the area between your shoulder blade and spine. Bring your shoulder back to neutral. Repeat four times.

Notice how your chest opens in the front as you draw your shoulder backward. You may even feel the abdominal muscles relax in the front.

Now move your shoulder in a slow, clockwise circle, drawing it first up to your ear, then arching it forward, then drawing it down in the direction of your waist, then slowly drawing it backward and up. Repeat this movement four times. Then reverse direction: move your shoulder in a counterclockwise circle—first up, then backward, then down, then forward and back to neutral again. Repeat the counterclockwise movement four times.

NOTICE AND SENSE

Notice whether it's easier to go forward or backward. Where does the circle become straight and not round? Does the movement feel smooth or jumpy? Slow it down, and smooth it out. Work without straining, but be aware of what you're doing.

For the movement in steps A–E, remember to slowly and gently contract, then lengthen and release the muscles. You're teaching those "frozen," tight shoulder muscles to "thaw out," and relax again. Each time you do these movements, your muscles will become a bit softer and more relaxed. Remember: it was movement that got you into the problem in the first place, so movement must get you out of it.

Standing Somatics

In Hanna Somatics, as in certain other forms of somatic education, we encourage people to lie on the floor to practice their movements. The reasoning behind this is that your brain will instantly, and in most cases, involuntarily instruct your body to engage in old patterns of muscular holding when you're standing up, or "in gravity." If you've got sensory motor amnesia, working on the floor is the most effective first step to retraining your muscles. Old habits can be changed—and new sensations felt—when you're not battling gravity. After doing your movements on the floor, you may feel different, strange, or out of balance when you stand up. These are words my clients use to describe the changes they feel once they begin to regain control of their bodies. But as soon as they become accustomed to the new sensations, the feeling of abnormality quickly disappears.

Once you've mastered the movements in the beginning of this book, and have achieved a greater range of mobility and balance in your back, waist, abdominals, neck, shoulders, and hips, there's no reason why you shouldn't stand up and practice some easy, fun, and functional movements designed to more deeply ingrain the good habits you've already learned. Break a habit *out* of gravity, and the new pattern is easier to integrate into your daily routine.

I created several of these movements for clients who wanted something they could do several times a day—almost anywhere—to remind them of how they wanted to feel: relaxed, long, stretched out, and balanced. We all reach up for things, reach across our desks, move our hips when we dance (if not, go sign up for a dance class—you'll be glad you did!), and move our shoulders and hips in opposition to each other when we walk. So why not turn these activities into an opportunity for strengthening your somatic education?

I'm convinced that incorporating standing somatics into one's daily routine can dramatically improve body awareness and freedom of movement. It's important to find something that you do every day that can be made into a somatic movement—whether it's walking upstairs, picking up the laundry basket, or lifting your children. Functional movement creates balanced, strong muscles that coordinate properly. So find a minute while you're waiting at the post office or train station and "reach up to the top shelf" to elongate your waist muscles and relax your whole body. Shift your hips up and down as if you're doing the salsa with an invisible partner. Why not? People might stare, but they also might join in the fun.

22

Reach Up to the Top Shelf

This movement is not only good for relaxing and lengthening the muscles at the core of your body, but it also serves a useful function in your daily life. Who hasn't had to "reach up to the top shelf" to get something? This standing version of the Human X (page 75) also relaxes the muscles in the front of your body.

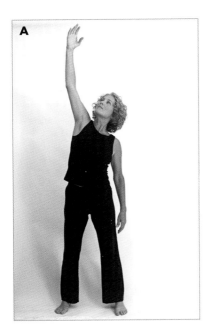

A. Stand in a neutral position on the floor or mat with your legs about hip width apart and with your hands at your sides. Reach your right arm up over your head as far as is comfortable. Look up at your hand. The right side of your ribs will open and your waist will get long.

Reach Up to the Top Shelf *(continued)*

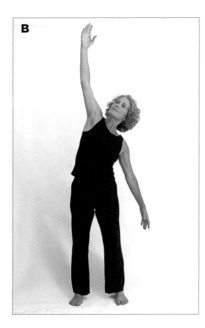

B. Without changing the position of your head, right arm, or right shoulder, reach down with your left arm. The left side of your ribs will contract and you'll get shorter in your waist on the left side. Now reach your right arm farther up and your left arm farther down at the same time.

Repeat the movement on the other side: reach your left arm up as far as is comfortable, then reach your right arm down as far as is comfortable. Notice any difference in your ability to reach up on the left side compared to the right side. Remember, it's the noticing that allows your brain to make more rapid changes in your muscles. Keep these sensations in mind as you move on to the next step of this movement.

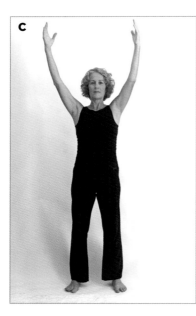

C. Keeping your head in a neutral, forward-looking position, bring both arms up above your head. Notice the length in both sides of your waist.

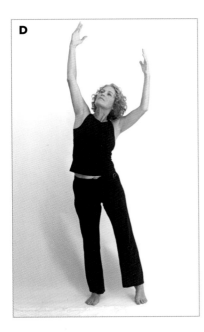

D. Reach your right arm up as if you were reaching for something you want to grasp. As you reach, push up onto the ball of your left foot, which will allow your left hip to slide upward. The left side of your ribs will squeeze down as the right side of your ribs opens.

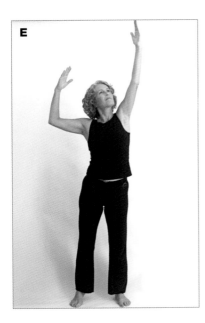

E. Return your right arm to neutral and reach your left arm up as if you were trying to grasp something. Let your right hip hike up as your right heel lifts off the floor. Both legs remain straight, and the left side of your ribs opens as the right side of your ribs squeezes down.

Repeat this movement several times, reaching up first with the right arm, then with the left arm. Make the movement as smooth as possible.

Reach Up to the Top Shelf *(continued)*

NOTICE AND SENSE

Just as with the Human X movement, notice how one side of your body shortens and the opposite side lengthens when you reach upward. The reaching comes not just from your shoulder, but also from the muscles deep in your back and waist. Notice the movement of your rib cage as you reach up with one side and let the other side squeeze. The movement is coming from the center of your body. You're lengthening and relaxing your back and waist muscles as you move through this pattern.

Let your hips move as you reach, and notice your hips the next time you really do have to reach up to the top shelf to get something. Follow through with this pattern of movement—involving your foot, hip, waist, ribs, and shoulder—and you'll be amazed at how high you can reach!

23

Diagonal Reach

This movement addresses the muscles involved in twisting and reaching. It will help you stay long through the center of your body, and also challenges your balance, because it involves shifting from one foot to the other.

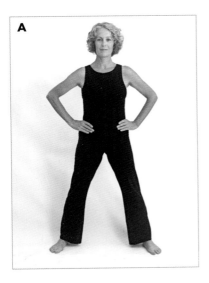

A. Stand with your feet slightly wider than hip width apart, and place your hands on your hips.

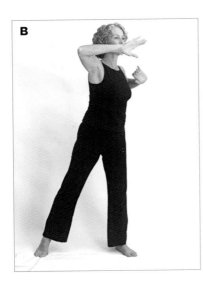

B. Bend both elbows and bring your hands in front of your chest, palms out. "Wing" your elbows out to the side. As you bring your left hand down, reach with your right arm diagonally across your body and up to the left, above your left shoulder. You will shift your weight onto your left leg as you do this, coming up onto the ball of your right foot.

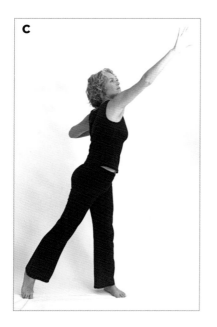

C. Straighten your right elbow and reach up as far as is comfortable, allowing your right leg to lengthen and your weight to come solidly onto your left foot. The upward reach comes from deep in the right side of your back. Notice the twisting of your torso as the left side of your body shortens. This is similar to the "reach to the top shelf" movement, only the reach is on the diagonal.

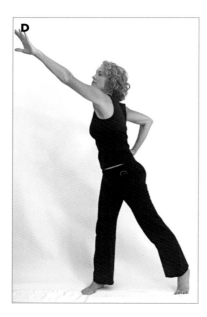

D. Now come back to neutral and then do the same movement on your left side: reach with your left arm across your body and up to the right. Let your weight come onto your right foot as your left leg straightens. Your torso twists, and your right shoulder pulls back as your left arm and shoulder reach up and forward.

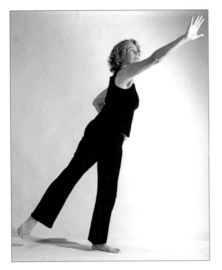

Variation

Once you get the feel of this movement, challenge yourself to balance on your standing leg and take your other foot off the floor for a second or two. If you're reaching up to the left, you'll pick up your right foot. If you're reaching up to the right, you'll lift your left foot off the floor. See how long you can balance!

NOTICE AND SENSE

Notice how one shoulder draws back as your other shoulder and arm reach forward. Sense the length in your back and waist as you twist across and up. Imagine you're throwing something high up into the air. Your hips and shoulders are twisting gently in opposition to each other. This opposition occurs naturally when we walk.

24

Reach Across

This movement, like the one before it, addresses the muscles of twisting and reaching, but it also incorporates more movement in the hips. Being able to pivot and turn is an important skill to maintain as we get older. This movement will help you stay grounded in your feet, which helps develop better balance.

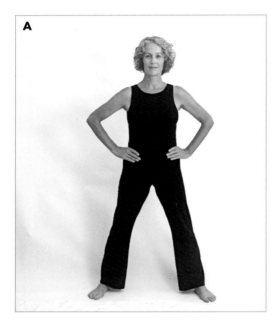

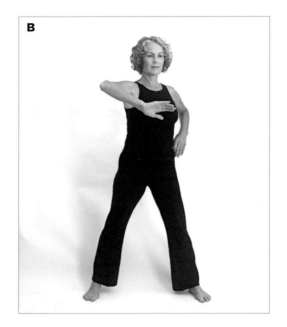

A. Stand with your feet slightly wider than hip width apart, and place your hands on your hips.

B. Leaving your left hand on your hip, bend your right elbow and bring your right hand in front of your chest, palm out. "Wing" your elbow out to the side. Reach with your right arm across your body, at chest height, to the left.

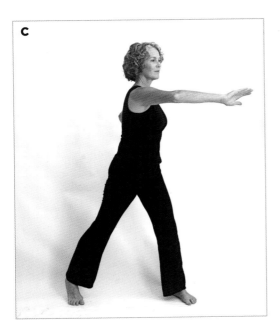

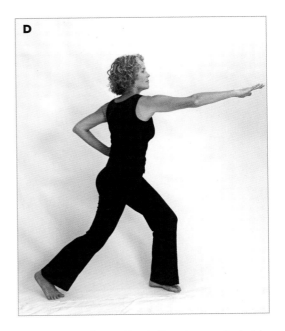

C. As you reach, allow your pelvis and right leg to turn as your foot pivots. Follow your arm with your head and your eyes. Allow your right foot to roll up until you're poised the ball of your foot.

D. Reach as far to the left as is comfortable and bend your knees. Your torso twists and your left shoulder pulls back as your right arm and shoulder reach across.

Reach Across *(continued)*

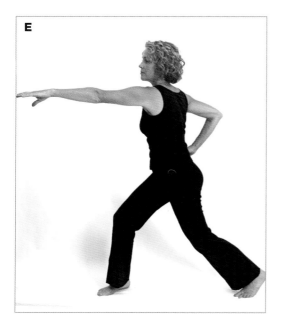

E. Now come back to neutral and then do the same movement on your left side: reach with your left arm across your body to the right. Allow your left hip and leg to pivot in the same direction. Follow your arm with your head and your eyes. Allow your knees to bend and your left foot to roll up. When you get comfortable with this movement, feel free to bend the knees further. This will help you feel more stable while also helping to strengthen your thigh muscles.

NOTICE AND SENSE

As you turn and reach, remember to allow your entire body—arm, shoulder, pelvis, leg, knee, and foot—to turn together. Make sure your knees are over your toes and that you have equal weight on both feet as you gently bend your knees. Sense the length in your back and waist as you twist across.

25

Hip and Shoulder Rolls

This standing movement simulates an important element of walking: the shoulders and hips moving in opposition to each other. It's a challenge, but it's fun. It's not unlike a movement you'd learn in dance class! The action of moving the shoulder and hips in opposition is common to jazz, swing, and ballroom styles of dancing.

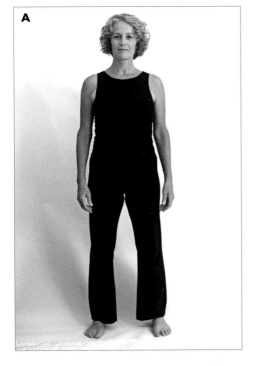

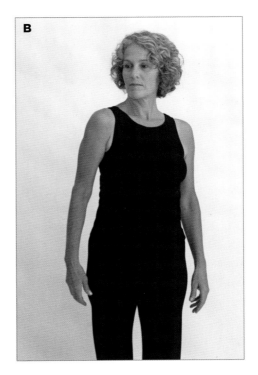

A. Stand in a neutral position on the floor or mat with your legs about hip width apart and with your hands at your sides.

B. Roll your right shoulder forward and notice how your left shoulder pulls back.

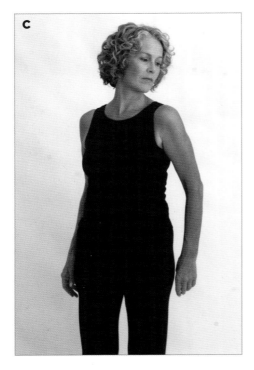

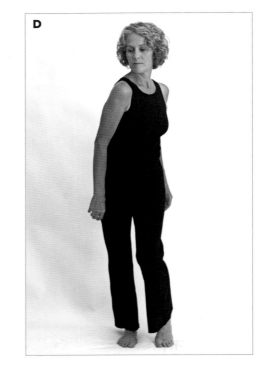

C. Now roll your left shoulder forward as your right shoulder pulls back.

Repeat steps B–C several times slowly.

D. Now let's combine your shoulders with your legs. Slowly roll your right shoulder forward as you bend your left knee. Let your foot roll up onto the ball of your foot as your left knee bends. Your left hip will hike up a little bit.

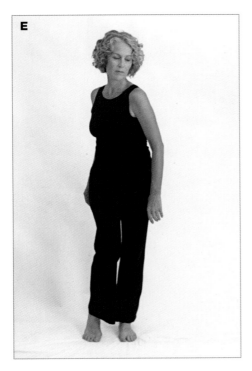

E

E. Now come back to neutral and then do the same movement on your left side: slowly roll your left shoulder forward, and at the same time slowly bend your right knee, rolling up on the ball of your right foot. Your right hip will hike up. Keep your left leg straight as you do this.

NOTICE AND SENSE

Do this movement slowly and gracefully. It follows the pattern of the Diagonal Arch and Curl (page 56)—one shoulder and elbow reaching toward the opposite knee and hip. Sense the diagonal contraction at the center of your body as you roll and contract your shoulder inward while reaching the opposite hip and knee forward. After you've gotten the hang of this pattern, you can put on your favorite music, add some arm movement, and start dancing!

26

Hip Rocking

This simple movement reminds you that as one side of your body lengthens, the other shortens—and that it all comes from the back, waist, and hips. Like hip and shoulder rolls, this movement is common to many dance styles; the hip roll is especially prevalent in merengue, rumba, and salsa.

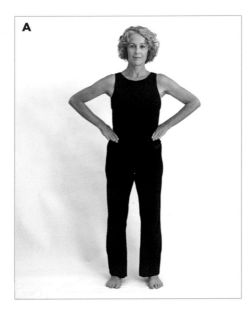

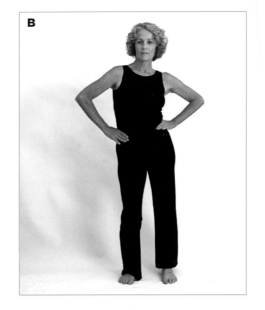

A. Stand with your feet at about hip width apart, and place your hands on your hips.

B. Bend your right knee and allow your left hip to hike up. Keep your left leg straight.

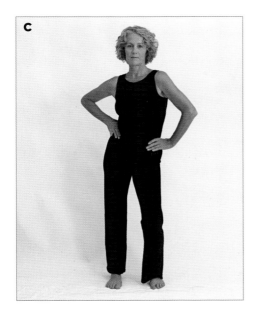

C. Now bend your left knee and allow your right hip to hike up as you straighten your right leg.

Repeat steps B–C several times. Get into a smooth rhythm: one knee bends, the other straightens. One hip hikes as the other relaxes.

NOTICE AND SENSE

This is the same pattern as found in the Human X (page 75) and Reach Up to the Top Shelf (page 113) movements: one side of the body is long and open as the other side shortens. You can also do this movement with both knees bent.

27

Getting to Know Your Feet

Ah, the feet! They're often neglected when it comes to movement. We usually focus on everything except our feet, which, as it happens, are an integral part of our balancing system. When we encase our feet in shoes, we risk losing both sensory awareness and motor control of all the muscles that help our feet turn in and out, flex and extend.

By the way, alert readers might notice that the lovely feet in the photographs on pages 128–131 aren't mine: they belong to my daughter, who has always taken good care of her feet and enjoyed walking barefoot.

She and I recommend that you spend some time playing with your feet. Begin by standing barefoot on a hard surface with your weight on both feet. Close your eyes and take a few minutes to sense your feet. What do they feel like? Is your weight resting more on the outside or the inside of your feet? Is your weight resting more on your heels or on the balls of your feet? Are your toes relaxed?

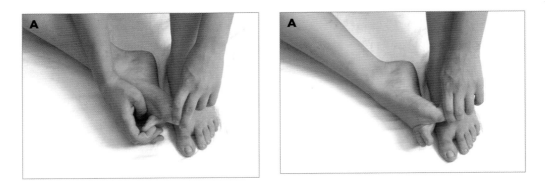

A. Sit on the floor and, using one or both hands, move the big toe on your right foot gently up and down. Notice how far up your foot the sensation travels. Be gentle!

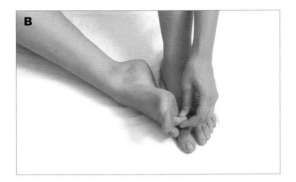

B. Do the same thing with your second toe—move it up and down. You're just exploring, like a baby playing with its toes!

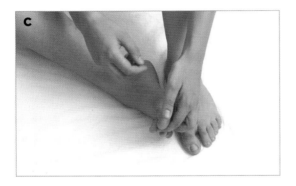

C. Go to the third toe and further explore the movement of up and down. Pull one toe up and the other down. Wake the toes up gently.

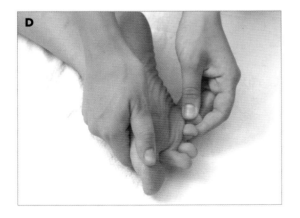

D. Do this with each individual toe until you get to the pinky toe.

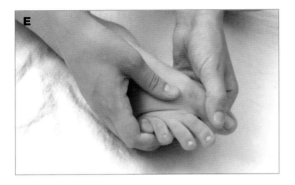

E. Next, pull your big toe in one direction as you gently pull the other toes in the other direction.

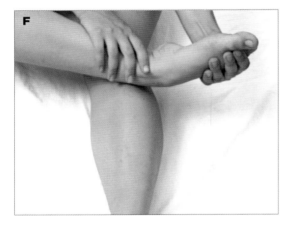

F. Cross your foot over your leg and gently use your hands to point your foot.

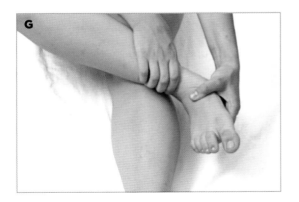

G. Use your hands to flex your foot, moving it only as far as is comfortable.

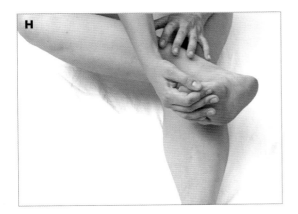

H. Use your hands to flex your toes. Notice the difference between flexing your entire foot and flexing just your toes.

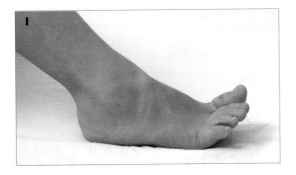

I. Place your foot on the floor and flex just your toes without lifting the ball of your foot.

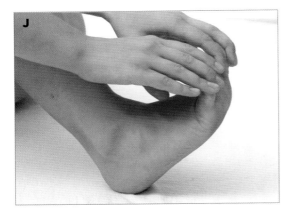

J. Keeping your heel on the floor, use your hands to flex your foot at the ankle, but add toe flexion as well. Gently pull your toes back.

Now stand up. Close your eyes and center your awareness on the foot you've just finished exploring. What does it feel like now? Let your brain soak up all the sensory feedback. Wiggle your toes if you like. Notice the difference in sensation between the foot you've just played with and the other foot. Repeat steps A–J on your left foot.

Getting to Know Your Feet *(continued)*

NOTICE AND SENSE

After you've completed the movements on both feet, stand up and compare the two. Does one foot feel the same as the other? If not, how do they feel different? Are you standing with your weight more centered than it was before you began the movement? Do you feel more aware of your feet? Take a walk around the room and sense the movement of your feet. Are you walking any differently, now that your feet are more awake?

Notice how the movement of your foot affects the muscles of your leg. Sense how the flexion of your foot causes your lower leg to contract. Notice your calf muscle as you point your toes. This is a powerful sequence that can really wake up tired, painful feet. Try to find a few minutes every day to play with, stimulate, and use your feet! This will greatly improve your balance.

I would suggest doing all standing somatics movements barefoot, if you can. Incorporate awareness of your feet into the movements. Notice how your feet ground you in the movement and provide stability.

Touch Your Toes

Most hamstring stretches are painful. They can often cause injury as well. That's why I didn't call this movement Stretch Your Hamstrings—after all, simply using your body weight to pull yourself down to touch your toes, and thereby stretch your hamstrings, just doesn't work. Why not? Because you're not actively engaging the brain to lengthen the muscles involved.

This movement, on the other hand, is a hamstring pandiculation, which requires you to pay attention to the muscles that tighten when you reach your limit. They're the same ones you need to recontract slightly, and then slowly release and relax, in order to get more length in the hamstrings. Don't forget that hamstring flexibility is aided by release and length in the extensor muscles of the back as well.

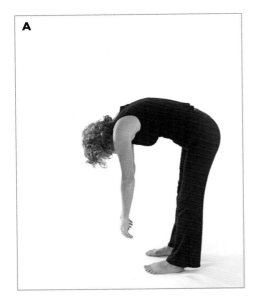

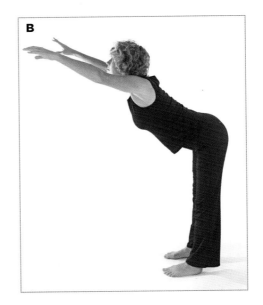

A. Let's test your present range of motion: reach down to touch your toes, without bending your knees. Let's say that you can only get as far as shown in the photo. What should you do?

B. Inhale, then lift your head, tighten your back, buttocks, and hamstrings, and lift yourself up a little.

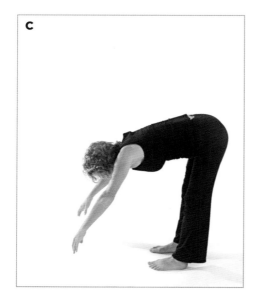

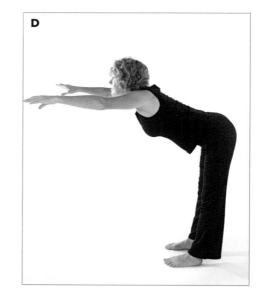

C. As you exhale, slowly release and lengthen down toward the floor as far as is comfortable. Then inhale and slowly lift your head again and tighten your back, buttocks, and hamstrings.

D. Again, slowly lengthen yourself down toward the floor as you exhale, only going as far as is comfortable. You will notice that it's easier to go farther down, as your muscles are being released actively. When you've gone as far as you can, inhale, lift your head, tighten your back in a bit of an arch, and engage your buttocks and hamstrings.

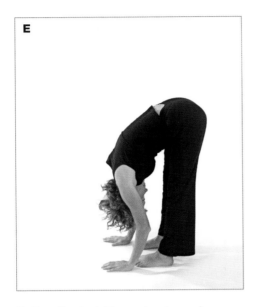

E. For the last time, slowly and consciously lengthen and release yourself down toward the floor as you exhale. See how far you've come!

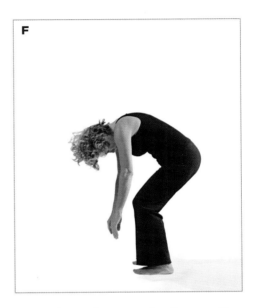

F. Bend your knees and roll yourself back up to a standing position, raising your head last.

Variation

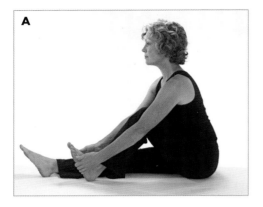

A. Sit up on the floor or mat with your left leg bent at the knee and your right leg straight out in front of you. Lift the toes of your left foot off the floor so that the heel of your foot is firmly planted.

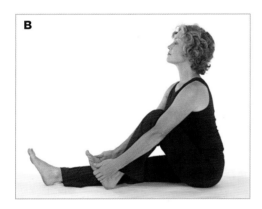

B. Inhale and gently pull the heel of your left foot back toward your buttocks as you straighten your back, tightening your back muscles slightly. Add some resistance with your hands so that your foot is pushing into your hands.

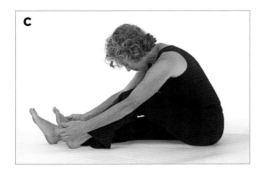

C. Slowly begin to straighten your left leg as you allow your back muscles to relax. Slowly drop your torso over your leg. Go about six inches or so and stop.

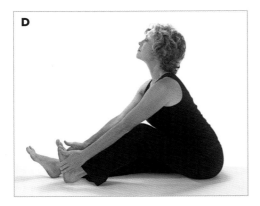

D. Reverse direction and tighten your leg back into your hands as you draw your foot back up a few inches. Tighten and straighten your back slightly and lift your head.

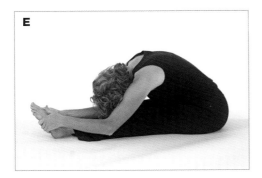

E. Slowly lengthen your leg again as you drop your torso, releasing your back muscles along the way. Go to your comfortable limit and completely relax.

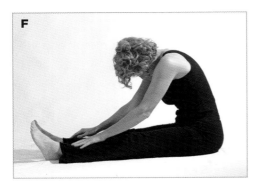

F. Slowly roll your torso up to neutral, making sure your head is raised last.

Touch Your Toes *(continued)*

NOTICE AND SENSE

By contracting your hamstrings and back first, then lengthening and releasing them, your range of motion increases. When you hit your limit, recontract your hamstrings and back, then release out a bit farther. As always, only go as far as is comfortable. If you think of this movement as a yawn—contracting first, then "yawning" the muscles out before you completely relax—it will get easier with every repetition. Because you're pandiculating both the hamstrings and your back muscles together as a coordinated unit, they should both feel relaxed and long.

PART III

Taking the Next Steps

More About Hanna Somatics

Hanna Somatic Education (also known as Clinical Somatic Education) may be defined as neuromuscular movement reeducation, the goal of which is to teach people to regain control of their sensory motor systems and in so doing improve the function and structure of their bodies and achieve better control of their movements. Simply put, Hanna Somatics teaches you to engage your brain (the command center of your muscles) in order to become aware of your body in space and the way in which you move—which in turn affects your muscles, joints, coordination, and balance.

Hanna Somatics directly addresses the relationship between the nervous system and the muscles, and the voluntary control the former has over the latter. It also teaches you to become aware of how you adapt to stress—either reflexively, as in a trauma, or habitually, as in repetitive movement. These adaptive responses to stress can hinder our movement and adversely affect our health. The more aware you are of your muscular system, the more power you have to change and control your body.

One-on-One Work

There are approximately 120 certified Hanna Somatic Educators worldwide. These somatic educators are trained to teach movement classes and conduct one-on-one, hands-on private sessions. Private sessions are geared toward teaching you to improve your internal awareness of movement: you learn to recognize which reflexive patterns you are stuck in (Red Light, Green Light, Trauma Reflex) and then to methodically release the sensory motor amnesia within those muscles. In computer speak, it's akin to hitting the Refresh button: eventually, new patterns will take the place of old patterns. Somatic educators don't fix people—they teach people to fix themselves.

For most people, just doing the exercises in this book will hone their proprioceptive skills and result in dramatic changes in muscle tone, coordination, balance, pain relief, and overall ease of movement. However, there are those for whom private, hands-on Hanna Somatics sessions are beneficial, especially those who have extreme pain or tightness, or deep, long-term postural misalignments that need detailed attention.

You have seen that the movements in this book focus on specific muscle groups within movement patterns in order to build awareness and motor control gently, slowly, and deliberately—rather like peeling away the layers of an onion, only from the inside out. So it is with private sessions. The somatic movement patterns in this book reflect the sequence of "homework" assignments in private sessions. Each movement reinforces the progress made in the previous session, thus incrementally improving flexibility, reducing pain, and increasing self-awareness. The more you do your somatic movements, the more self-aware, self-monitoring, and self-correcting you will become and the less likely you will be to suffer a recurrence of your previous muscular problems.

Afterthoughts

Over the past several years, I have had the privilege of spending time in India and Africa on more than one occasion. A friend reminded me of something I had written upon my return from my first visit to India, which I share as food for thought.

I have several observations about "somatic India": first, walking slowly and not driving cars or sitting at computers for hours on end can help relieve painful, tight hips. In addition, squatting to go to the bathroom is good for you (as long as both knees are strong)! It relaxes the back, opens the hips, tones the core, and lets everything go. I saw no Red Light Reflex to speak of in India— just balanced posture . . . Walking everywhere—and I don't mean rushing—really makes you aware of how we seem to *attack* every-thing we do in America. We have so much, yet we're always rushing to do something else, something more. Many of us seem to live in a "fight or flight" state of mind . . . Sitting on the floor instead of in a chair can make an amazing difference in joint flexibility. You have to move around frequently while on the floor, so it keeps you from getting stuck in one position. In one school I visited there were no desks or chairs, so the children sat on the floor while they did their lessons. Moving was allowed, not discouraged. Sometimes I was left wondering whether I was looking at the past or looking at what I hope the future will be.

There has been very little clinical research directed toward somatic education, perhaps because of the fact that somatic education isn't medical. This lack of research is unfortunate, because somatic education is one of the most effective and inexpensive methods by which certain functional problems—such as chronic back pain, neck and shoulder pain, sciatica, or plantar fasciitis—can be addressed successfully for the long term. Does surgery succeed in curing certain cases of back pain? In certain traumatic situations, the answer would have to be yes. But ultimately, muscles learn to contract due to commands from the brain, and it is somatic education—brain reeducation—that achieves the longest-lasting results.

I echo Thomas Hanna's assertion that if we could teach our children, from a very young age, to maintain sensory motor awareness of their bodies, we could prevent perhaps hundreds of thousands of cases of musculoskeletal pain and dysfunction that cost our health-care system billions of dollars. Hanna observed that children aren't *taught* hand-to-eye coordination, nor are they *taught* to crawl. They learn these skills through direct experience. They spend the first several years of their lives, after all, doing nothing but exploring their bodies and their environment. Then they go to school, where they are encouraged to sit still and keep their eyes on the blackboard, so that gradually they learn to ignore themselves internally in order to focus externally. Although external focus is a useful and necessary skill, children are often punished for being physical in the classroom. They are taught to be acute in their distance perceptions and hearing, but to ignore the internal awareness of their bodies.

Once we lose the ability to learn through direct experience, though, we begin to lose our flexibility, our movement, our balance. It's a case of use it or lose it.

I am convinced that somatic education is one of the most important and effective ways to promote and preserve the health and longevity of our generation and those to come. It is a field in health care whose time is now. It's about returning people to a natural state of physical awareness and autonomy. Whether or not you choose to work with a somatic educator, you can learn to reverse your muscle pain, improve your movement, and live a more active and physically fulfilling life simply by practicing the movements and principles in this book. After all, as Thomas Hanna once told his students, "There is no one who will care as much about you as *you*."

Sample Routines for Your Daily Somatics Practice

While it is best to do a longer Somatics practice each day, below you will find some sample routines to choose from when time is limited. These sessions may be abbreviated, but you will still address all the major muscles of your body so that you will start, and end, your day with more aware, relaxed, and controlled muscles.

5 minute routine:
- Arch and Flatten
- Arch and Curl
- Washrag
- Reaching to the Top Shelf

10 minute routine:
- Arch and Flatten
- Arch and Curl
- Washrag
- Walking Exercises

15 minute routine:
- Arch and Flatten
- Back Lift
- Arch and Curl
- Washrag
- Walking Exercises
- Reaching to the Top Shelf

30 minute routine:
- Arch and Flatten
- Arch and Curl
- Back Lift
- Cross Lateral Arch and Curl

- Side Bend
- Washrag
- Human X
- Steeple Twist
- Seated Twist
- Walking Exercises
- Reaching to the Top Shelf

60 minute routine:
- Go through all the movements in the book, beginning with Arch and Flatten, and ending with the Posture Pillow Exercise for walking.

Once you learn the movements in this book, you can be creative with your routine. Remember, however, to begin slowly and build your routine to include one movement for the back of the body, another for the front of the body, another for twisting or side bending, and another for movement of the pelvis. Experiment! You'll find that many of these movements can even be done while seated.

Enjoy your daily practice! Put time aside for yourself, even if you can only spare just five minutes each day. Regular focused movement, which involves both body and brain, will help you keep the mobility and suppleness you need for pain-free living—no matter your age.

Resources

Websites

Association for Hanna Somatic Education—www.hannasomatics.com: the professional association for Hanna Somatic Educators

Exuberant Animal—www.exuberantanimal.com: Frank Forencich's website for books, workshops, Exuberant Animal trainings, and ideas for fun, vigorous play-based fitness.

Hooping Harmony—www.hoopingharmony.com: a website that sells handmade hoops and hooping products—Greenfield, MA

Luna Sandals—www.lunasandals.com: simple sandals for runners and others who want to go barefoot without going barefoot.

Movetheory—www.movetheory.com: a site by Dr. Kwame Brown that discusses the Move Theory. Move Theory engages with individuals and organizations throughout the United States to create Active Play for children and adolescents.

MovNat: Explore Your True Nature—www.movnat.com: MoveNat is a system of functional and natural movement training based on the movement skills that helped humans adapt on earth.

Soft Star Shoes—www.softstarshoes.com: a great place to buy shoes designed for natural movement and healthy feet (soft-soled moccasins, shoes, and slippers for children and adults).

Sparkinglife—www.sparklinglife.org—the website of author and professor psychiatry Dr. John Ratey. This site is about exercise and its positive effect on brain development.

Books

Alon, Ruthy. *Mindful Spontaneity: Lessons in the Feldenkrais*. California: North Atlantic Books, 1996.

Doidge, Dr. Norman. *The Brain That Changes Itself: Stories of Personal Triumph from the Frontiers of Brain Science*. New York: Penguin Books, 2007.

Feldenkrais, Moshe. *Awareness Through Movement: Easy-to-Do Health Exercises to Improve Your Posture, Vision, Imagination, and Personal Awareness*. New York: HarperCollins, 1977.

Forencich, Frank. *Change Your Body, Change the World: Reflections on Health and the Human Predicament*. Washington: Exuberant Animal, 2010.

Forencich, Frank. *Exuberant Animal: The Power of Health, Play, and Joyful Movement*. Indiana: AuthorHouse, 2006.

Forencich, Frank. *Play As If Your Life Depends On It: Functional Exercise and Living for Homo Sapiens*. Washington: GoAnimal, 2003.

Hanna, Thomas. *Bodies in Revolt: A Primer in Somatic Thinking*. California: Freeperson Press, 1970.

Hanna, Thomas. *The Body of Life: Creating New Pathways for Sensory Awareness and Fluid Movement*. Vermont: Healing Arts Press, 1979.

Hanna, Thomas. *Somatics: Reawakening the Mind's Control of Movement, Flexibility and Health*. Massachusetts: De Capo Press, 1988.

Jamison, Kay Redfield. *Exuberance: The Passion for Life*. New York: Vintage Books, 2004.

John, Dan. *Never Let Go: A Philosophy of Lifting, Living and Learning*. California: On Target Publications, 2009.

Ratey, Dr. John, and Eric Hangerman. *Spark: The Revolutionary New Science of Science and the Brain*. New York: Little, Brown and Company, 2008.

Index

About the Author

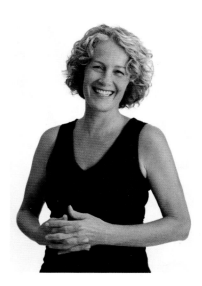

Martha Peterson is a Certified Hanna Somatic Educator who has worked for three decades in the field of movement. She is a former professional dancer, and has a BA in Dance Education and professional certification in Hanna Somatic Education from the Novato Institute for Somatic Research in Novato, California. She teaches Hanna Somatics both privately and in group classes, both in her studio in Maplewood, New Jersey, and internationally. She works with people of all ages who suffer from chronic pain and disability due to back, neck, hip, and shoulder pain, scoliosis, TMJ (temporomandibular joint disorder), Carpal Tunnel Syndrome, and repetitive use and sports injuries. Martha is an avid hiker and traveler, and lives with her family in Maplewood, New Jersey.